COLOUR GUIDE

Oral Pathology

R. A. Cawson MD FRCPath FDS
Emeritus Professor of Oral Medicine and Pathology, University of London, UK
Visiting Professor, Baylor University Medical Center and Dental College, Dallas, Texas, USA

E. W. Odell FDS PhD MRCPath
Senior Lecturer in Oral Medicine and Pathology, United Medical and Dental Schools of Guy's and St Thomas's Hospitals, University of London, UK

SECOND EDITION

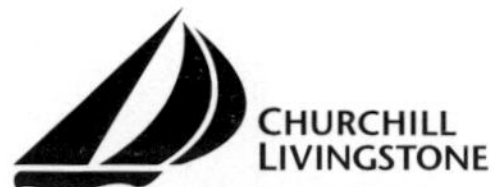

CHURCHILL LIVINGSTONE

EDINBURGH LONDON NEW YORK PHILADELPHIA ST LOUIS SYDNEY TORONTO 1999

CHURCHILL LIVINGSTONE
A Division of Harcourt Publishers Limited

First published as Colour Aids—Oral Pathology, 1987
First Colour Guide edition 1993
Second Colour Guide edition 1999

ISBN 0443 06171 8

British Library of Cataloguing in Publication Data
A catalogue record for this book is available from the British Library.

Library of Congress Cataloging in Publication Data
A catalog record for this book is available from the Library of Congress.

Medical knowledge is constantly changing. As new information becomes available, changes in treatment, procedures, equipment and the use of drugs become necessary. The authors and the publisher have, as far as it is possible, taken care to ensure that the information given in this text is accurate and up to date. However, readers are strongly advised to confirm that the information, especially with regard to drug usage, complies with current legislation and standards of practice.

The publisher's policy is to use **paper manufactured from sustainable forests**

Printed in China
SWTC/01

For Churchill Livingstone

Publisher: Michael Parkinson
Project editor: James Dale
Design: Eric Bigland
Project controller: Nancy Arnott

Preface to the second edition

We have taken the opportunity to add even more photomicrographs and to improve others wherever possible. Within the constraints of the format we have also tried to re-order the subject matter more rationally. The text has also been completely updated but, in view of its brevity, this Colour Guide should be used in conjunction with a fuller text such as *Essentials of Oral Pathology and Oral Medicine.*

London
1999

R.A.C.
E.W.O.

Contents

1 / Developmental defects of teeth

Aetiology

Genetic
- Amelogenesis imperfecta—hypoplastic or hypocalcified types
- Dentinogenesis imperfecta

Acquired
- Rickets
- Severe metabolic disturbances
- Fluorosis
- Tetracycline pigmentation

Microscopy

Amelogenesis imperfecta
- *hypoplastic type*—defective matrix formation—enamel irregular, overall thin, sometimes nodular or pitted but well-calcified, hard and translucent (Fig. 1).
- *hypocalcified type*—normal matrix formation and morphology but soft and chalky, and readily chipped away.

Dentinogenesis imperfecta: mantle (superficial) dentine with regular tubules; remainder—a few irregular tubules, inclusion of small blood vessels (Fig. 2). Enamel defects are also sometimes present.

Rickets: if severe can cause hypocalcification with a wide area of predentine and many interglobular spaces (Fig. 3).

Severe metabolic disturbances: typically affect enamel matrix producing linear pitting enamel defects corresponding to degree of tooth formation at time of illness.

Tetracycline pigmentation: teeth usually of normal form but stained yellow, degrading to grey or brown. Hard sections show yellow fluorescence along incremental lines under UV light (Fig. 4).

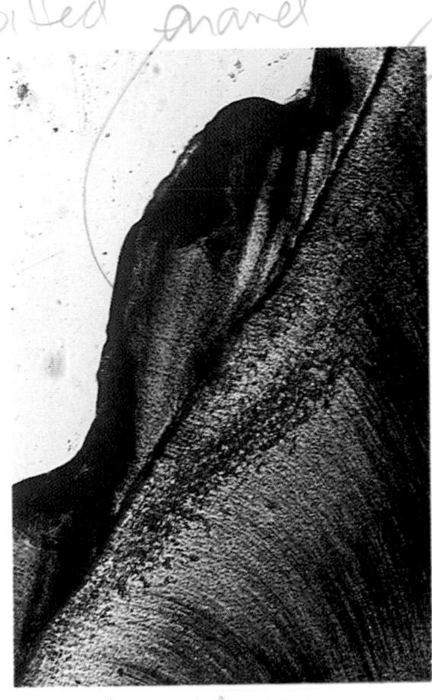

Fig. 1 Amelogenesis imperfecta: hypoplastic type.

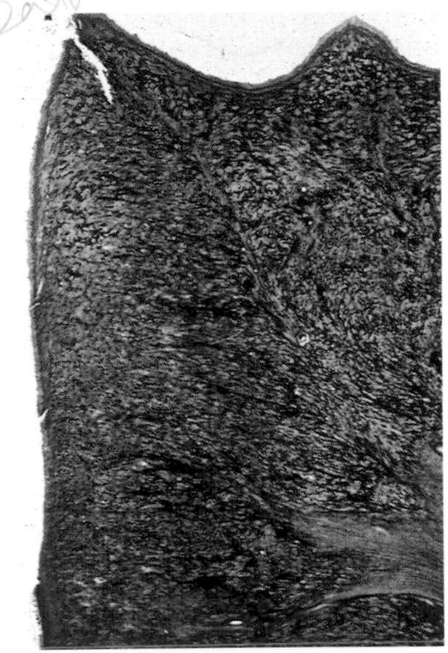

Fig. 2 Dentinogenesis imperfecta.

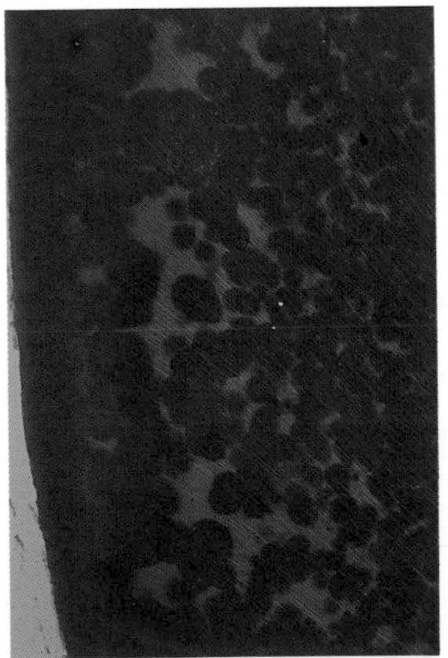

Fig. 3 Rickets.

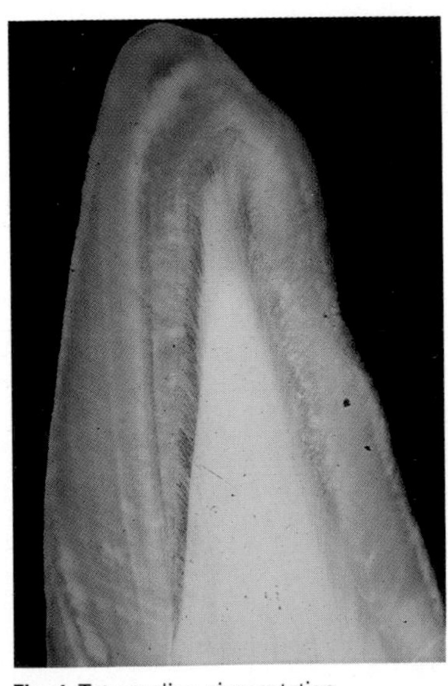

Fig. 4 Tetracycline pigmentation.

2 / Dental caries

Aetiology

- Bacteria: probably mainly acidogenic and glucan-forming strains of *Strep. mutans.* Other viridans streptococci, lactobacilli or actinomyces may contribute, possibly at different stages.
- Plaque: adherent meshwork of bacteria in polysaccharides, thickest in stagnation areas, concentrates bacterial acid production and delays buffering by saliva (Fig. 5).
- Susceptible tooth surface and (possibly) immune responses.
- Frequent supply of bacterial substrate—mainly sugar (sucrose).

Enamel caries

Microscopy

Pre-cavitation stage: bacterial acid leads to production of increasing size and numbers of submicroscopic pores in enamel.

Light microscopy shows conical area of change with apex deeply (Fig. 6), comprising:

- dense surface zone (more radiopaque) with enhanced striae of Retzius
- main body of lesion
- dark zone
- peripheral translucent zone.

Degrees of demineralization in different zones are assessed by polarized light studies and microradiography. Progressive demineralization eventually allows entry of bacteria.

Secondary enamel caries: bacteria reach and spread along the amelodentinal junction (Fig. 7) and attack enamel from beneath over a wide area. The term *secondary enamel caries* is also used for caries recurring beside restorations.

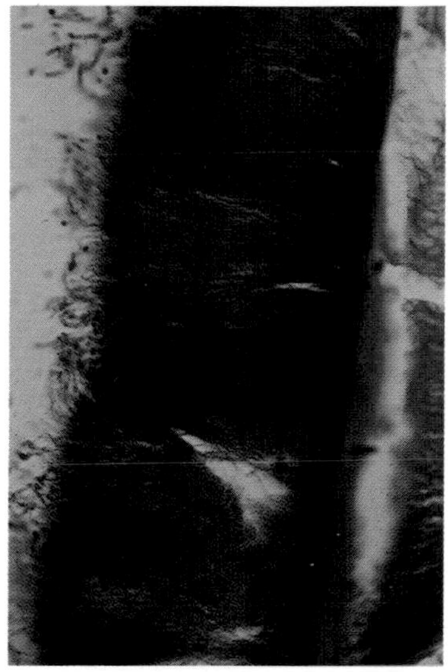

Fig. 5 Bacterial plaque on enamel surface.

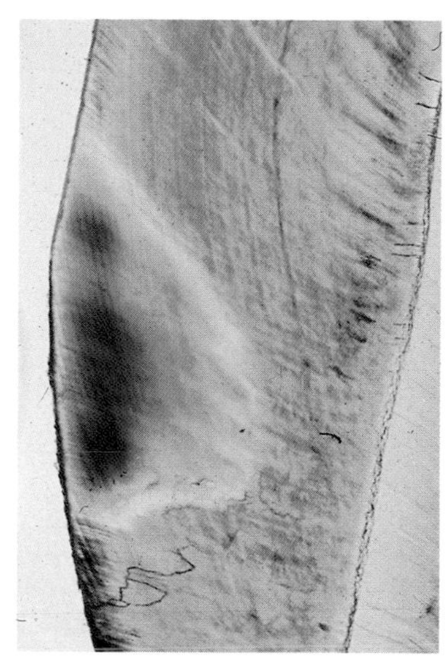

Fig. 6 Early caries (pre-cavitation stage).

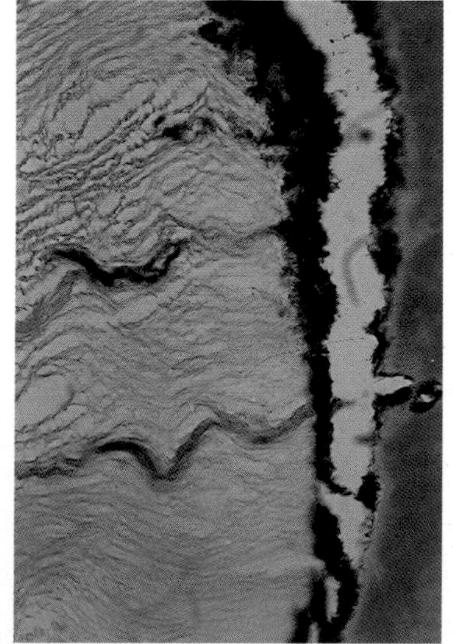

Fig. 7 Secondary enamel caries.

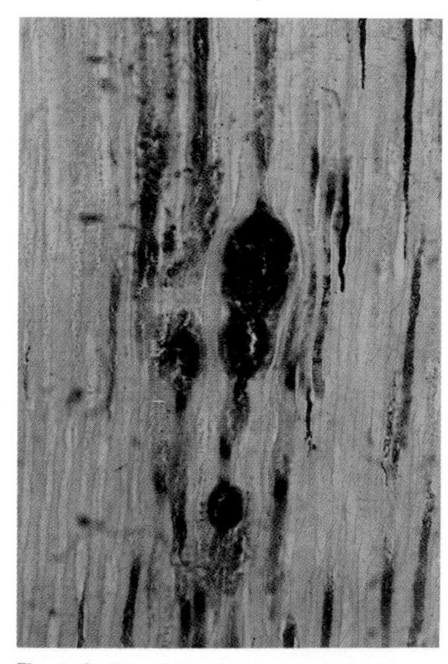

Fig. 8 Caries of dentine.

Dentine caries

Bacteria spread along the amelodentinal junction (see Fig. 7, p. 4) and down dentinal tubules. Softening of the matrix by bacterial acids causes distension of tubules (see Fig. 8, p. 4). Any dentine exposed by enamel destruction is colonized by plaque, which extends destruction over a wide area (Fig. 9).

Microscopy

Dentine is demineralized by bacterial acids from bacteria spreading along the amelodentinal junction and invades via the tubules, a conical lesion being formed.

Walls of tubules in softened dentine become distended by bacteria. Intervening dentine breaks down to form liquefaction foci (Fig. 10) and the tissue progressively disintegrates.

Dentinal reactions

Dead tracts

Odontoblasts are killed in acute caries and pulpal ends of tubules sealed off by calcified material.

Translucent zones

In very chronic caries or attrition, tubule walls become progressively calcified (peritubular dentine) until tubules are obliterated (Fig. 11).

Reactionary dentine

Regular tubular dentine forms under chronic lesions. Irregular dentine with few, irregular tubules forms beneath more acute lesions (Fig. 12).

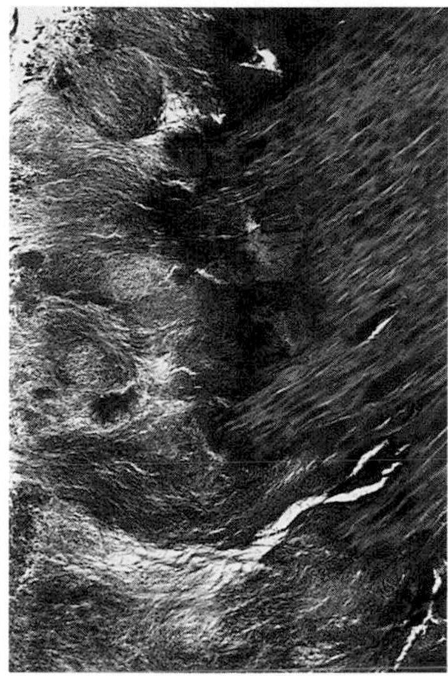

Fig. 9 Plaque invading dentine.

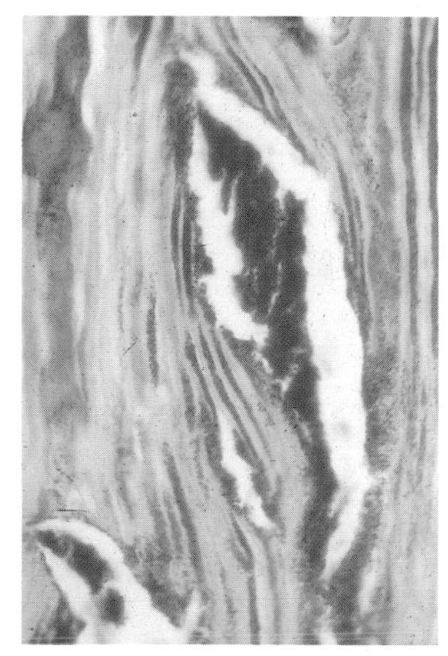

Fig. 10 Bacteria destroying dentine. (High power.)

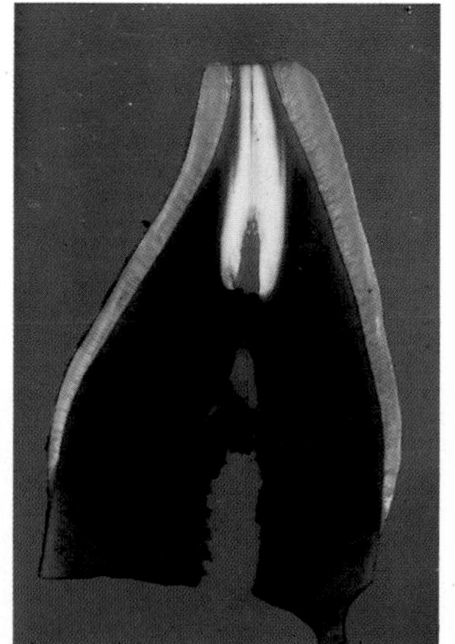

Fig. 11 Translucent zone.

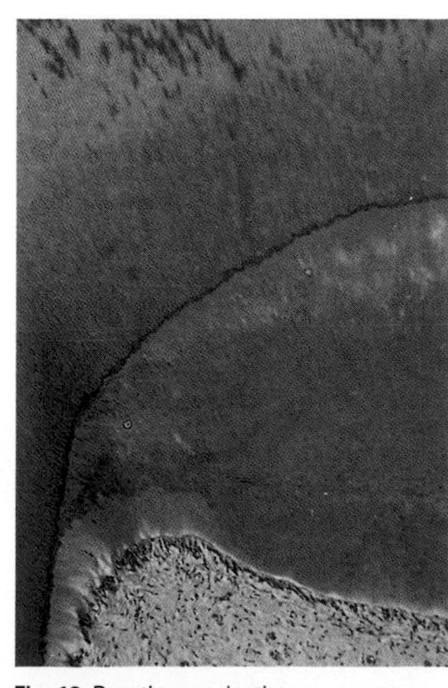

Fig. 12 Reactionary dentine.

3 / Pulpitis

Aetiology

- Caries (most commonly)
- Traumatic exposure (cavity preparation, fracture or cracked tooth)
- Thermal or chemical irritation, or both, from restorations

Closed pulpitis

Acute closed pulpitis

Typical inflammatory reactions are initially localized to a minute area (Fig. 13) but typically lead to necrosis of pulp due to restriction of blood supply at the apical foramen, compression of vessels by oedema in the confined space, and thrombosis.

Microscopy

All degrees of severity may be encountered, namely:

- acute hyperaemia and oedema (Fig. 14)
- progressive infiltration by neutrophils
- destruction of specialized pulp cells
- abscess formation (Fig. 15)
- cellulitis (Fig. 16)
- necrosis.

(There is little correlation between symptoms and histological picture but acute pulp pain is usually indicative of irreversibly severe pulpitis.)

Microscopy

Chronic closed pulpitis

- Predominantly mononuclear inflammatory cells (lymphocytes, plasma cells and macrophages).
- Initially localized pulp damage. Destruction of pulp is often relatively slow.
- Often an incomplete calcific barrier around inflammatory focus.
- Usually, necrosis of pulp eventually results.

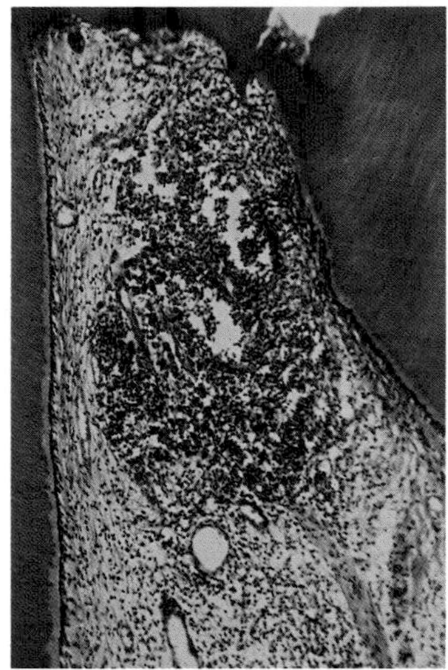

Fig. 13 Localized pulp abscess.

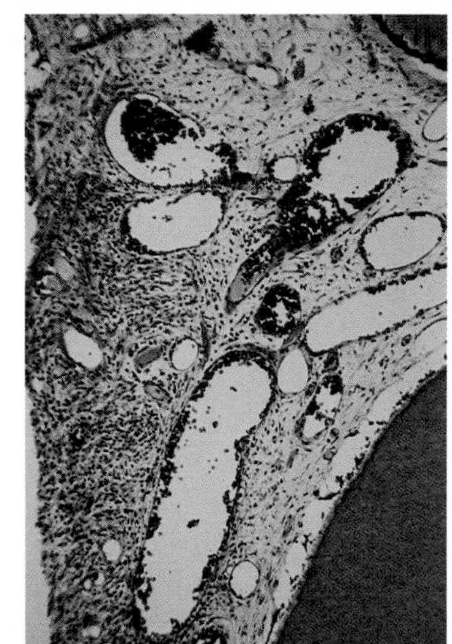

Fig. 14 Hyperaemia of pulp.

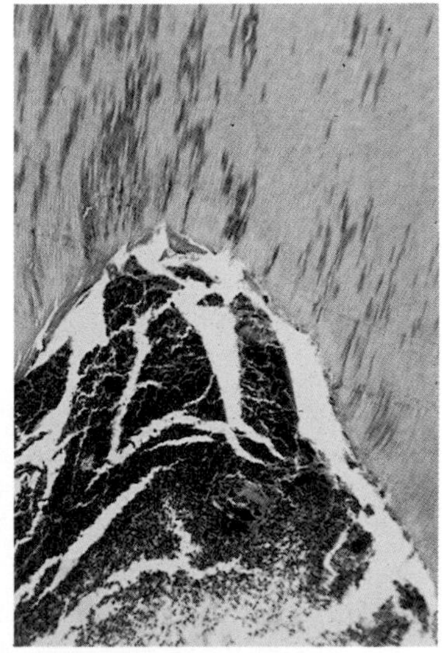

Fig. 15 Advanced pulp abscess.

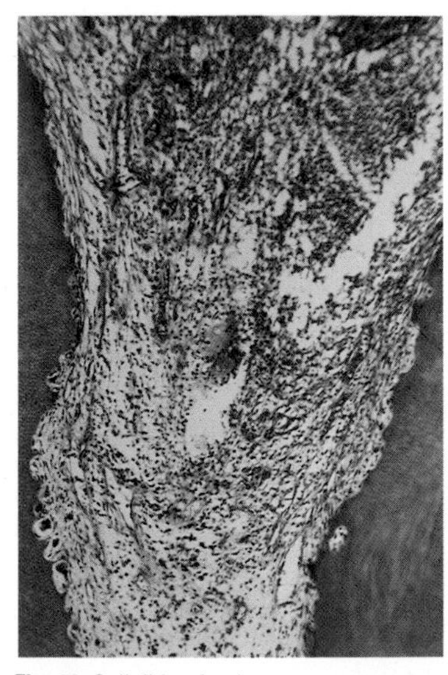

Fig. 16 Cellulitis of pulp.

Open pulpitis

Wide exposure of the pulp by carious destruction of the crown may allow it to survive by relieving the pressure of exudate. Survival of pulp in these circumstances may be more likely in teeth with open, incomplete apices. Inflammation extends throughout the pulp, which becomes replaced by granulation tissue (Fig. 17).

Microscopy

Granulation tissue may proliferate through the exposure and become colonized by epithelial cells. Proliferation of the epithelium may lead to the formation of an almost complete covering, allowing subsidence of inflammation beneath (except at the margins in contact with the edges of the carious dentine and plaque) and progressive fibrosis of the mass. The pulp polyp (Fig. 18) thus formed appears as a pink or red nodule protruding from a wide exposure. Destruction of nervous tissue in the mass renders it insensitive.

Other pulp changes

Calcification

- *Secondary to pulpitis.* Calcifications may form at the border of localized low-grade pulpitis and coalesce to surround it completely (dentine bridge). However, the bridge is permeable and inflammation extends beneath it (Fig. 19). Dentine bridges, seen on X-ray after pulp treatment, do not necessarily therefore indicate complete healing of the underlying pulp.
- *Diffuse granular calcification.* Fine calcifications may progressively extend through normal pulps and fuse to form large masses (Fig. 20). They are of no clinical significance.
- *Pulp stones.* Large calcified masses of tubular dentine may form in the pulp, some at least as excrescences from the walls. They are not necessarily age-related, and are seen in young persons with the dental abnormalities of Ehlers—Danlos syndrome. Pulp stones are asymptomatic; their chief significance is possible obstruction in root canal treatment.

Internal resorption: (see p. 13 and Figs 25–27, p. 14).

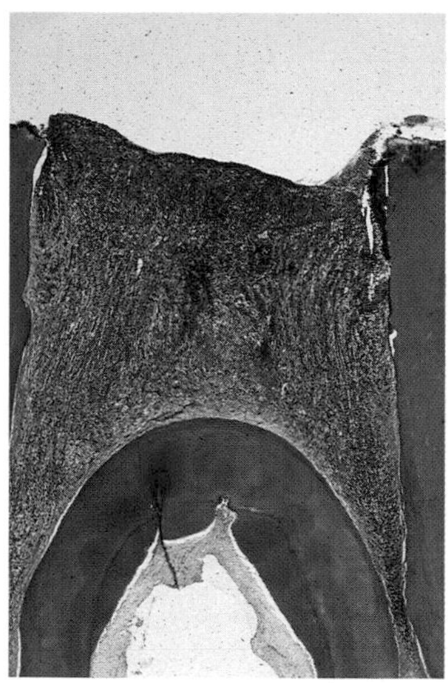

Fig. 17 Chronic open pulpitis.

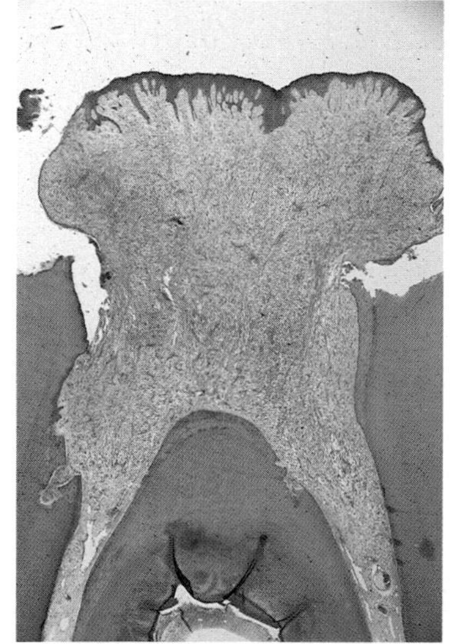

Fig. 18 Open pulpitis; epithelialized polyp.

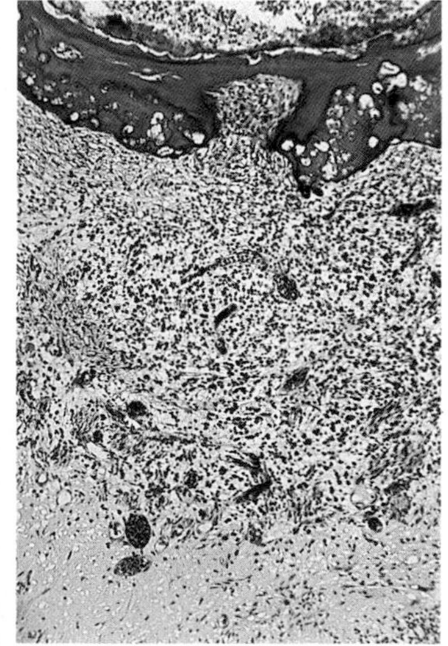

Fig. 19 Calcification ('dentine bridge') under pulpitis.

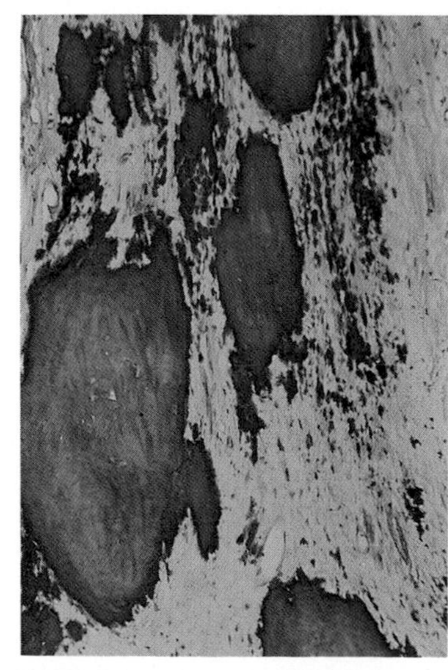

Fig. 20 Pulp stones and calcifications.

4 / Apical periodontitis

Aetiology

- Secondary to caries and pulp necrosis in most cases
- Trauma to tooth severing apical vessels
- Root canal treatment (irritant medicaments or overextension)

Microscopy

Acute: accumulation of acute inflammatory cells (neutrophils) and fluid exudate in potential space between apex and periapical bone (Fig. 21).
If neglected, there is suppuration and resorption, usually of buccal plate of bone, and sinus formation on the gum overlying the apex of the tooth. In deciduous molars, inflammation, often interradicular, i.e. overlying permanent successor, develops.

Chronic: low grade inflammation. Granulation tissue (fibroblasts and capillary loops) proliferates with varying density of inflammatory infiltrate.
A rounded nodule of granulation tissue (apical granuloma) forms, with resorption of periapical bone to accommodate it (Figs 22 & 23).

Epithelial content: rests of Malassez are often destroyed by inflammation. If not, they may proliferate (Fig. 24) in apical granulomas to form microcysts. The epithelial lining is variable in thickness. Eventually, a radicular cyst may thus form.

Pus formation: neutrophil infiltration and low grade suppuration usually lead eventually to discharge via sinus on gingiva or occasionally on skin over apex.

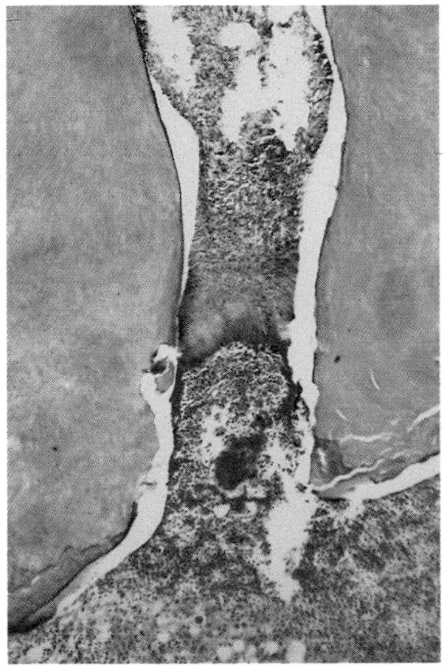

Fig. 21 Acute periapical periodontitis.

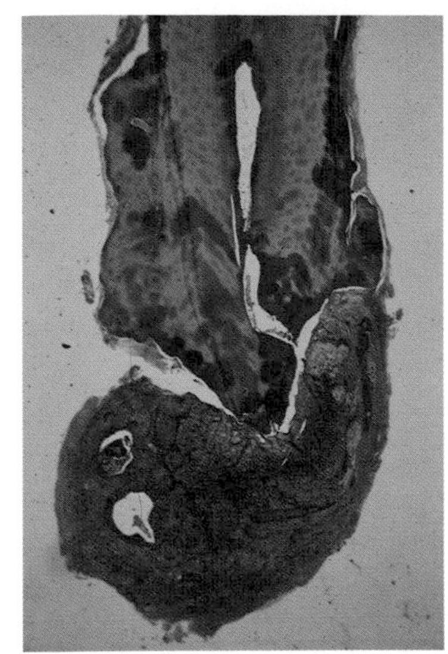

Fig. 22 Apical granuloma.

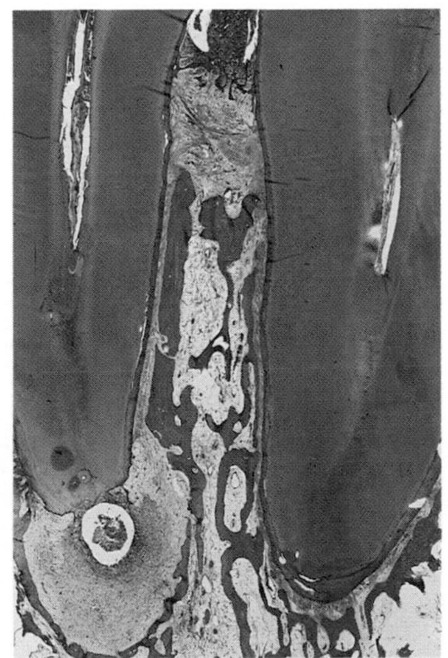

Fig. 23 Apical granuloma in situ.

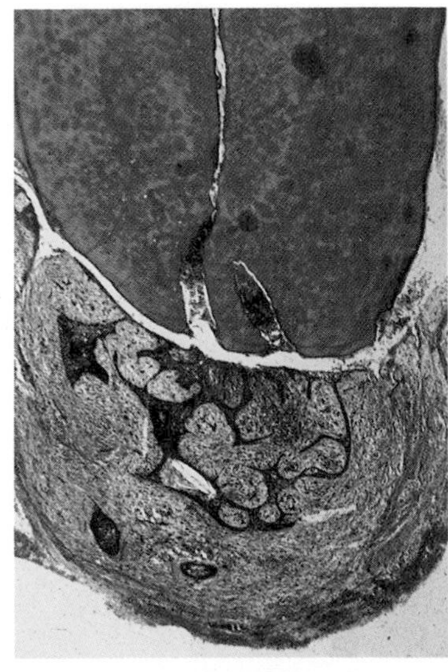

Fig. 24 Apical granuloma with epithelial proliferation.

5 / Resorption and Hypercementosis

Resorption

Aetiology

Normal: in deciduous teeth before shedding

Pathological:
- idiopathic—internal or external
- secondary (local inflammation, pressure from malposed tooth or tumour, orthodontic movement, replantation, buried teeth)

Microscopy

Idiopathic: progressive resorption by giant cells, mainly of dentine. There is sometimes intermittent reparative activity to form a complex pattern of resorption and bone-like reparative tissue. Resorption (internal or external) can expose pulp (Figs 25–27). Pulpitis follows.

Secondary: usually localized giant cell activity. Variable reparative activity with hard tissue deposition is seen.

Hypercementosis

Aetiology

- Ageing
- Chronic apical periodontitis (adjacent to resorption)
- Buried teeth, Paget's disease
- Cementomas (p. 53)

Microscopy

Usually lamellar—sequential deposition of layers of cementum forming smooth thickening of root. Rarely (Paget's disease or cementoblastoma), there is an irregular jigsaw-puzzle ('mosaic') pattern of intermittent deposition and resorption (Fig. 28).

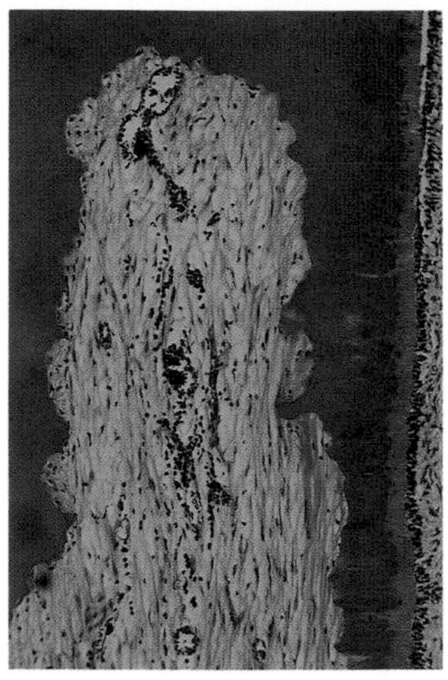

Fig. 25 Internal resorption of dentine.

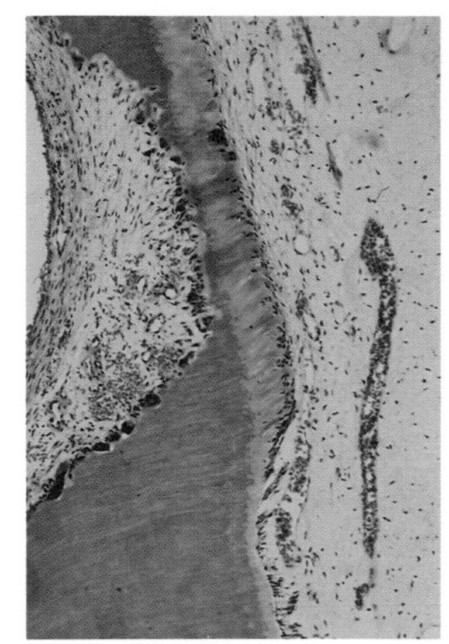

Fig. 26 External resorption.

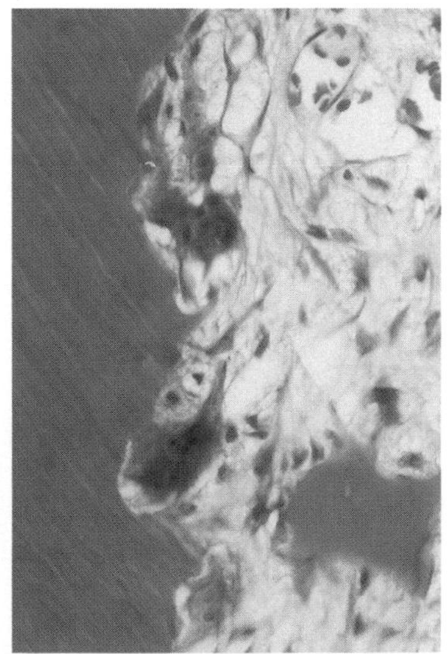

Fig. 27 Internal resorption showing giant cells.

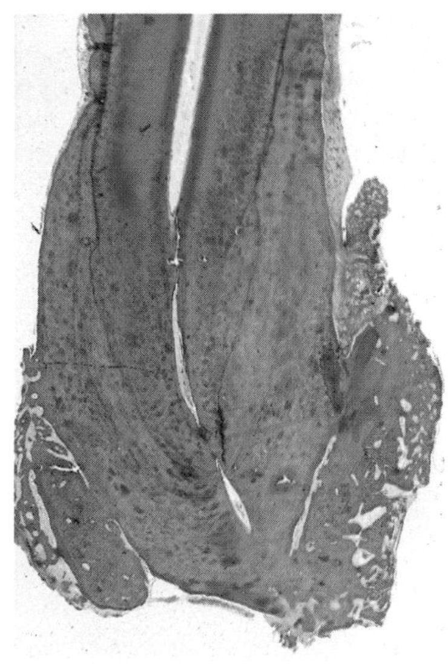

Fig. 28 Hypercementosis: lamellar and irregular.

6 / Periodontal disease

Normal periodontal tissues

Gingival epithelium comprises:

- *oral epithelium*—extends from mucogingival junction to crest of gingival margin and has rete ridges
- *sulcular epithelium*—joins the oral and junctional epithelia
- *junctional epithelium*—tends to be flattened and forms a union with the tooth in the epithelial attachment extending to the amelodentinal junction in normal mature tissue, apical to which is the periodontal ligament.

Connective tissue *gingival fibres* support the gingival margin as a cuff around the tooth. *Transeptal fibres* join adjacent teeth and, more deeply, *horizontal fibres* join the tooth to the socket wall (Figs 29 & 30 and Fig. 34, p. 18).

Acute ulcerative gingivitis

Aetiology

Otherwise healthy young adults affected. Aetiology unknown but is associated with:

- poor oral hygiene
- smoking
- upper respiratory tract infections
- stress.

Microbiology

Overwhelming proliferation of Gram-negative anaerobic bacteria traditionally termed *Fusobacterium nucleatum* and *Borrelia (Treponema) vincentii*. Other anaerobes may also be involved.

A smear shows this fusospirochaetal complex (Fig. 31) and polymorphs.

Microscopy

Gingival necrosis and non-specific ulceration covered by slough containing fusiforms and spirochaetes. Tissue is invaded by spirochaetes with progressive destruction of marginal gingivae (Fig. 32) and then of deeper supporting tissues. There is no generalized stomatitis.

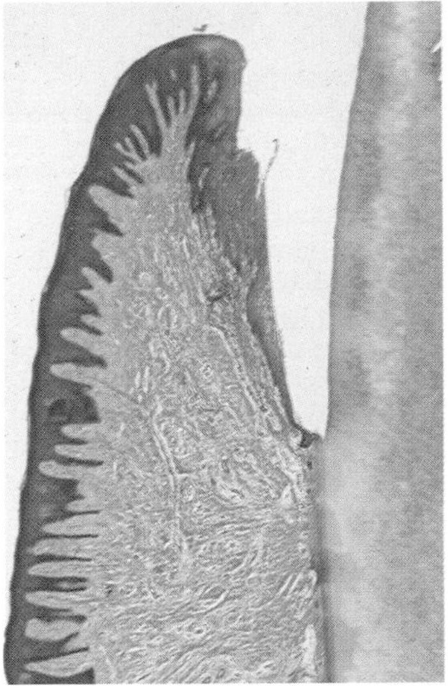

Fig. 29 Normal human adult buccal gingiva.

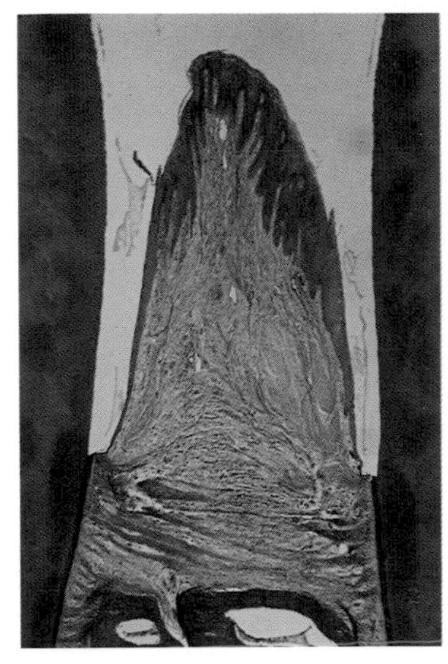

Fig. 30 Normal human adult interdental gingiva.

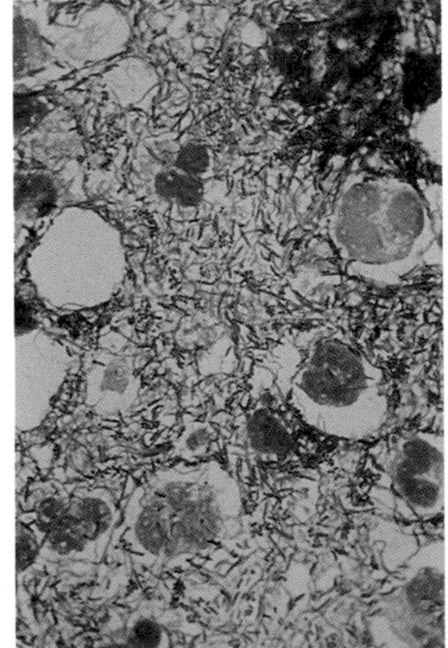

Fig. 31 Acute ulcerative gingivitis: fusobacterial complex in smear.

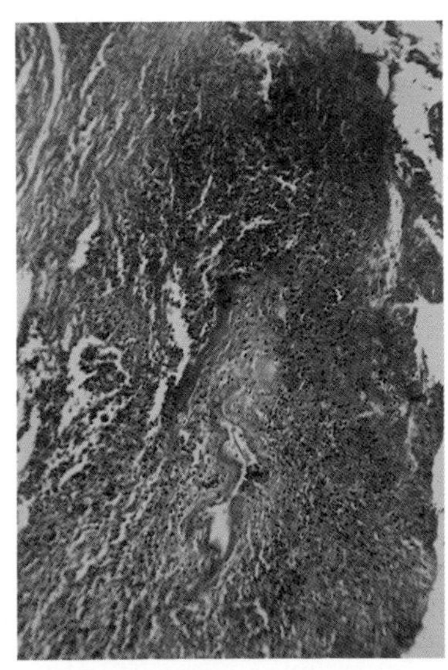

Fig. 32 Acute ulcerative gingivitis: gingival necrosis.

Chronic gingivitis

Aetiology

Inflammatory response to bacterial plaque accumulating at the gingival margin. The bacterial population is mixed with no specific pathogens identified although, initially, bacteria are Gram-positive and aerobic. An increasing bulk of plaque (100–300 cells thick) is associated with increasing prominence of Gram-negative bacteria, such as veillonellae, fusobacteria and campylobacter. The process is probably initiated by leakage of bacterial antigens from plaque in the gingival sulcus.

Microscopy

Plaque on tooth surface with inflammation sharply localized to vicinity of plaque. There is an initial hyperaemic stage (Fig. 33) with relatively scanty inflammatory cells in the corium. By definition, the periodontal ligament is not involved and the epithelial attachment to enamel persists despite inflammatory cells extending beneath it (Fig. 34). The inflammatory infiltrate becomes increasingly dense but is sharply confined to the marginal gingiva (Fig. 35). It is predominantly lymphoplasmacytic and the protective antibody response is shown by antibody production in plasma cells (Fig. 36).

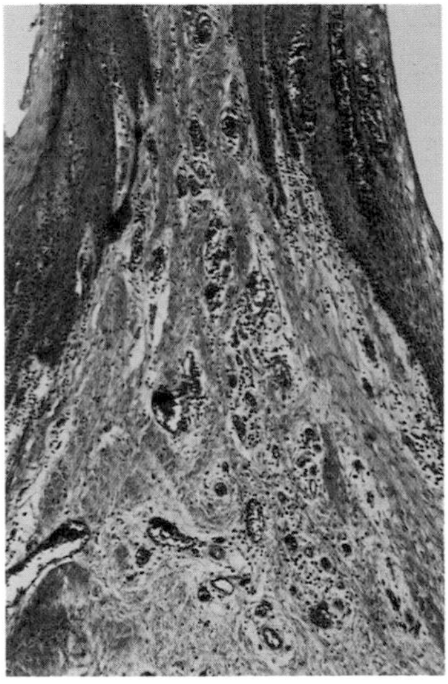

Fig. 33 Marginal gingivitis: early hyperaemic stage.

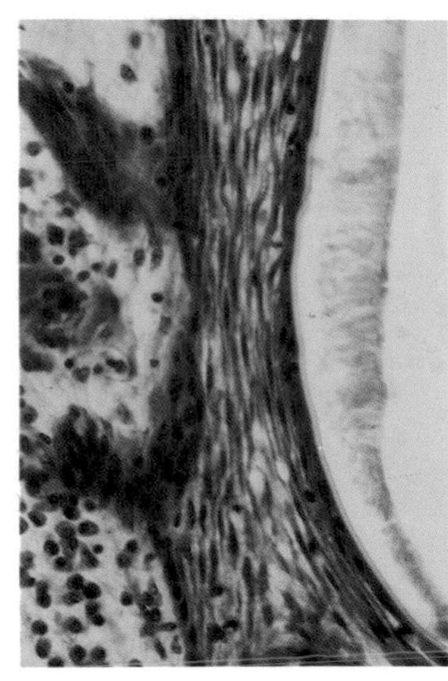

Fig. 34 Junctional epithelium and epithelial attachment on enamel in gingivitis.

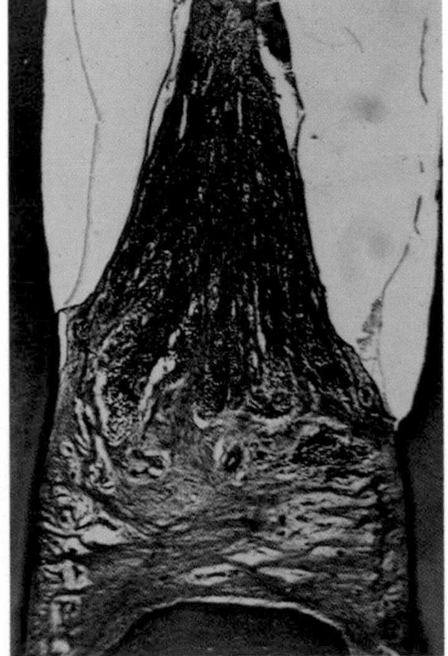

Fig. 35 Marginal gingivitis: dense chronic inflammatory infiltrate.

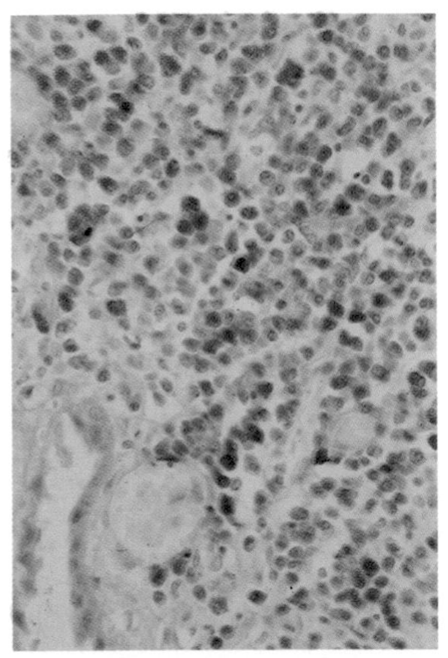

Fig. 36 Immunoperoxidase showing antibody production in plasma cells.

Chronic periodontitis

Aetiology

Persistence of bacterial plaque. Progression of inflammation with tissue destruction is a common but not invariable sequel to chronic gingivitis; there is wide individual variation for unknown reasons.

Microbiology and immunology

Many potent pathogens (e.g. *Porphyromonas* species, capnocytophaga, clostridia, fusobacteria, etc.) can be isolated from periodontal pockets, but individual roles in tissue destruction are uncertain. Some (e.g. *Actinomyces* species) produce bone resorbing factors. A defensive immune response (antibody production and cellular immunity) to plaque bacteria is detectable. Evidence of immunologically mediated tissue destruction is speculative only and not consistent with histological findings. Periodontal destruction is accelerated in immunodeficient patients but host factors affecting prognosis of periodontal disease have not been identified in otherwise healthy persons.

Microscopy

1. Plaque and often calculus on tooth surface extending into pockets (Figs 37 & 38).
2. Predominantly lymphoplasmacytic infiltrate in gingival margin and pocket walls, not extending more deeply and not involving alveolar bone (Figs 38 & 39).
3. Rootward migration of epithelial attachment (Fig. 40).
4. Destruction of periodontal ligament fibres and alveolar bone, but osteoclasts rarely seen.
5. Formation of epithelium-lined pockets with epithelial attachment in floor.

Gradual rootward progress of destruction leads eventually to loosening of teeth. Tissue destruction is usually uniform along the arch (horizontal bone loss) but local factors may promote more complex patterns of destruction. Localized destruction of bone around individual teeth (vertical bone loss) may develop or, occasionally, there is a more rapid destruction of periodontal ligament than alveolar bone with extension of pocketing between teeth and bone (intrabony pocketing).

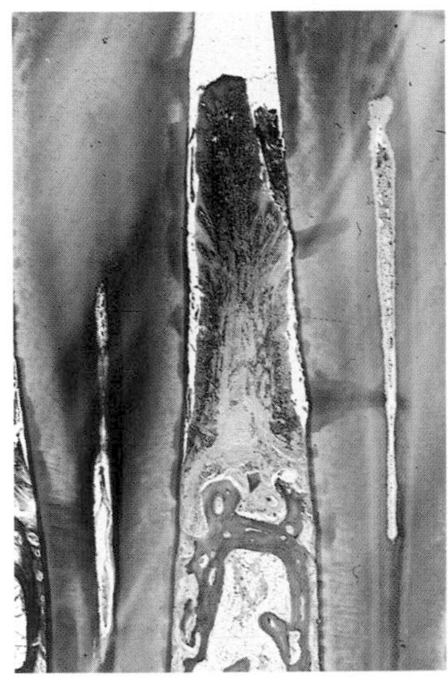

Fig. 37 Chronic periodontitis. Note inflammatory infiltrate localized to vicinity of plaque.

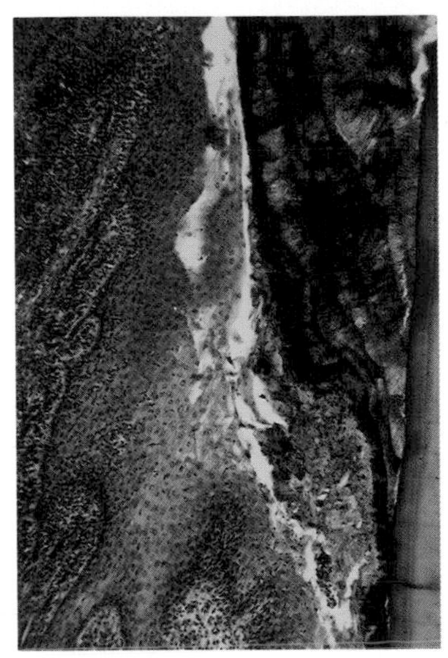

Fig. 38 Periodontal pocket: plaque and calculus, and epithelial lining.

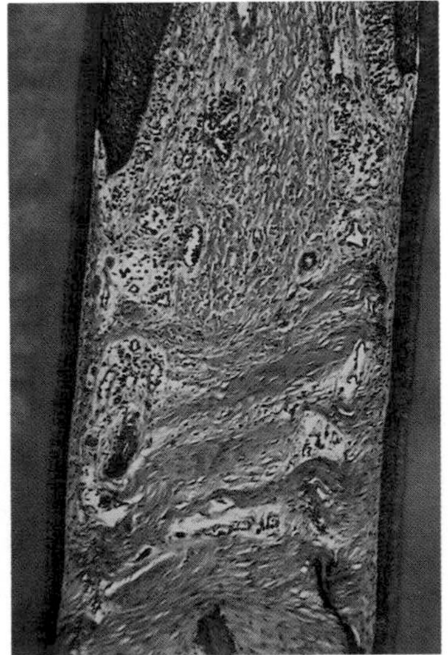

Fig. 39 Chronic periodontitis: inflammation-free zone between floor of pocket and bony crest.

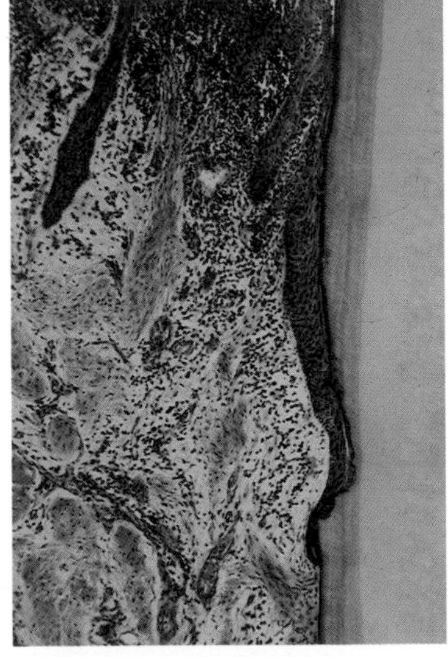

Fig. 40 Periodontitis. Migration of epithelial attachment along cementum.

Advanced chronic periodontitis

Destruction may progress until tooth support becomes inadequate and more complex patterns of bone loss develop (Fig. 41).

Intrabony pockets extend deep to the crest of the alveolar bone and are difficult to manage. Despite the deep extension of inflammation it may remain clear of the alveolar bone closely adjacent, which may also lack any sign of osteoclastic activity histologically (Fig. 42).

Periodontal (lateral) abscess

Aetiology

Usually a complication of advanced periodontitis. It may be due to injury to the pocket floor (?food-packing) or more virulent infection.

Pathology

- Rapid acceleration of periodontal destruction.
- Destruction of epithelial pocket lining.
- Dense neutrophil infiltrate and suppuration (Fig. 43).
- Widespread osteoclastic resorption of bone (Fig. 44) increasing width and depth of pocket to form deep intrabony pocket.
- Pus may exude from pocket mouth or point on attached gingiva.

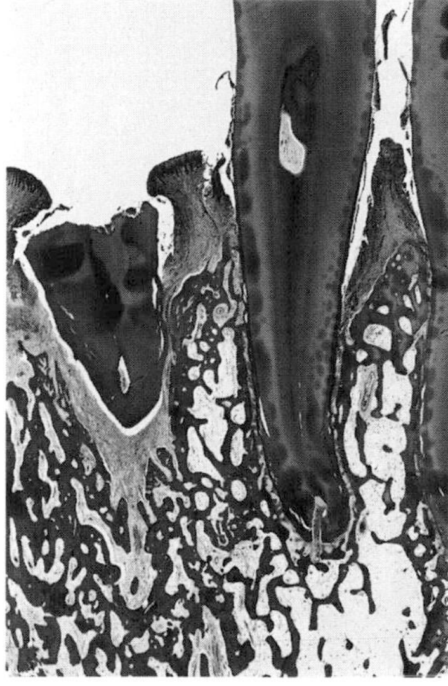

Fig. 41 Late periodontitis with intrabony pocket.

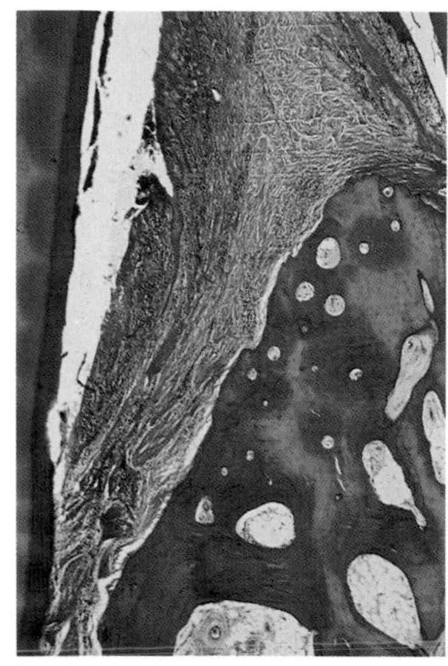

Fig. 42 Higher power view of intrabony pocket.

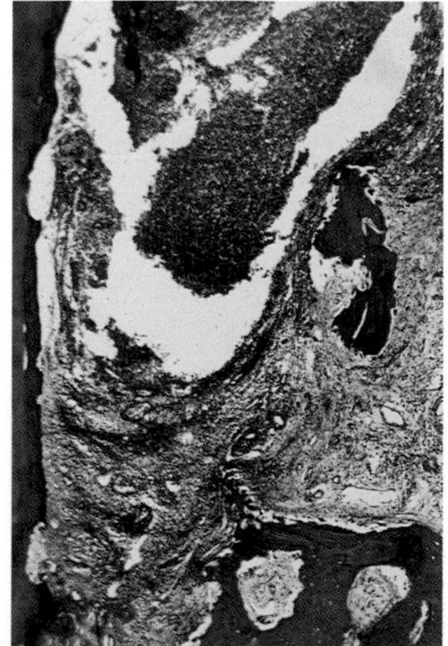

Fig. 43 Periodontal abscess.

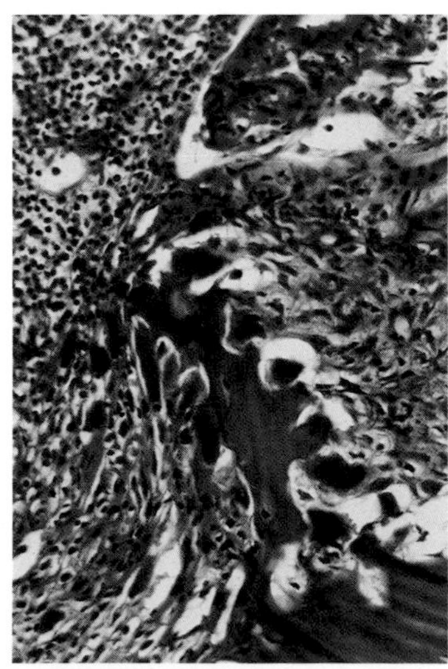

Fig. 44 Giant cells resorbing bony floor of periodontal abscess.

Gingival recession

Aetiology

- Wear and tear from over-vigorous toothbrushing
- Severe uncontrolled ulcerative gingivitis
- Some cases of chronic periodontitis

Microscopy

Gradual destruction of gingival tissue, periodontal ligament and bone, all at similar rates. No pocket is formed. There is low grade minimal chronic inflammation (Fig. 45).

Gingival swelling

Microscopy

Acute myelomonocytic leukaemia
Exaggerated response to plaque, with gross infiltration of gingivae by leukaemic cells, gingival swelling and accelerated periodontal destruction (Fig. 46).

Fibrous hyperplasia
Hereditary type: generalized smooth gingival swelling may overgrow and conceal erupting teeth.

Drug-associated hyperplasia: produces bulbous swellings of interdental papillae. Causes include phenytoin, cyclosporin, nifedipine and its analogues (calcium channel blockers).

Both show hyperplasia of gingival collagen with 'stretching' of elongated rete ridges (Fig. 47).

Pregnancy epulis (pregnancy tumour)
Consists of dilated thin-walled vessels in loose oedematous stroma often with superimposed inflammation (Fig. 48). The condition is not distinguishable from a pyogenic granuloma except by the pregnant state.

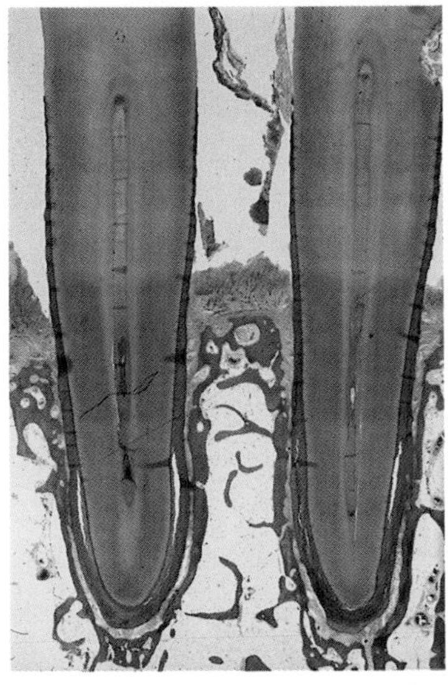

Fig. 45 Gingival and periodontal recession.

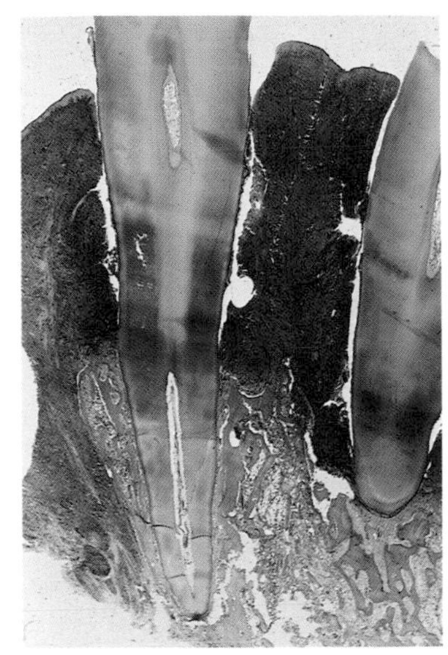

Fig. 46 Acute myelomonocytic leukaemia: gingival infiltration.

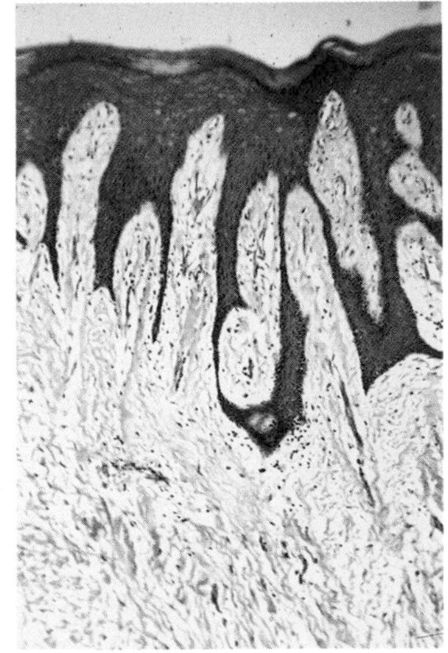

Fig. 47 Gingival fibromatosis.

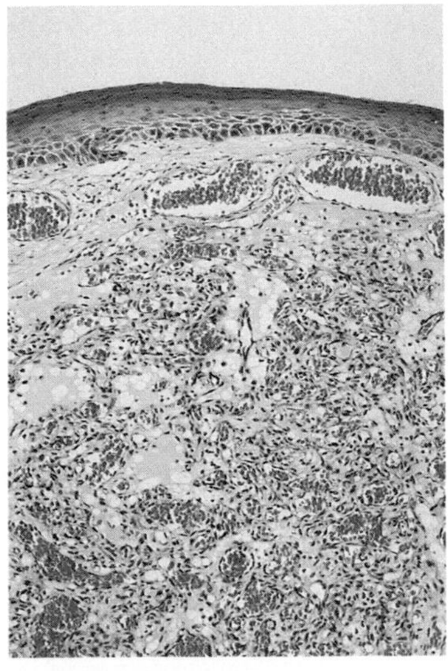

Fig. 48 Pregnancy epulis.

7 / Cysts of the jaws

Radicular cysts (1)

Aetiology

Pulp death, apical periodontitis, proliferation of epithelial rests of Malassez, cystic change in epithelium; expansion of cyst by hydrostatic pressure; resorption of surrounding bone.

Incidence

65–75% of jaw cysts. Radicular cysts are the most common types of cyst and cause of chronic swellings of the jaws.

Microscopy

Components comprise:

- epithelial lining
- chronic inflammatory infiltrate
- fibrous wall
- bony shell undergoing progressive resorption.

The epithelial lining is stratified squamous in type and very variable in thickness; sometimes with arcaded configuration (Fig. 49), irregularly acanthotic (Fig. 50) or, rarely, very thick (Fig. 51). In some areas, the epithelial lining may be destroyed (see Fig. 53, p. 28). The underlying inflammatory infiltrate is also of variable density. The fibrous wall allows enucleation of the cyst from its bony shell. Bone shows progressive resorption on the inner aspect and apposition externally (Fig. 52), but resorption typically outpaces apposition so that the lateral wall is eventually destroyed.

In the late stages, distension of cyst leads to thinning of the epithelial lining and, if infection is not superimposed, the inflammatory infiltrate becomes attenuated (Fig. 52).

Residual cysts

The causative tooth is extracted, leaving a residual cyst. They are typically found late in life, and show late-type features.

Lateral radicular cysts

These are rare and related to a lateral root canal of a non-vital tooth. ➡

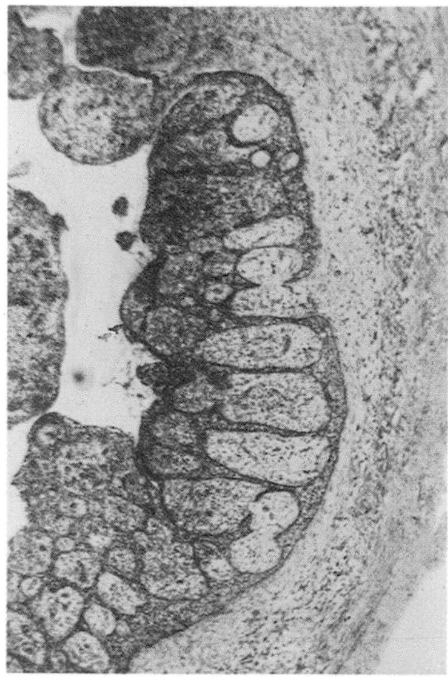

Fig. 49 Arcaded epithelium of cyst lining.

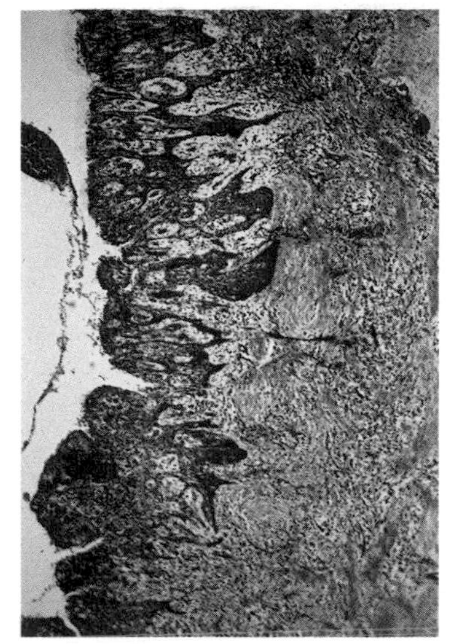

Fig. 50 Inflamed cyst with irregular epithelial lining.

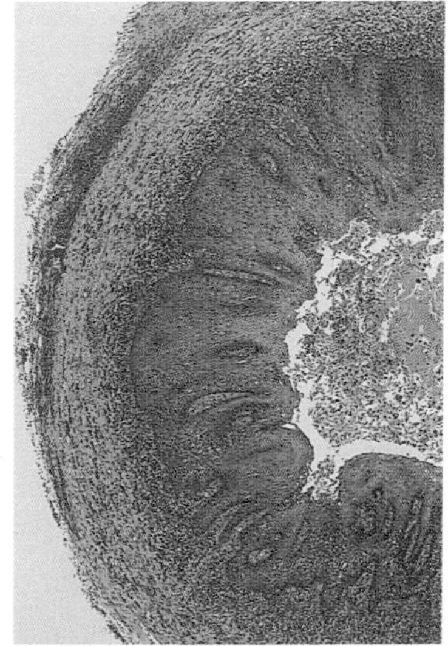

Fig. 51 Radicular cyst. In this example the epithelial lining is conspicuously hyperplastic.

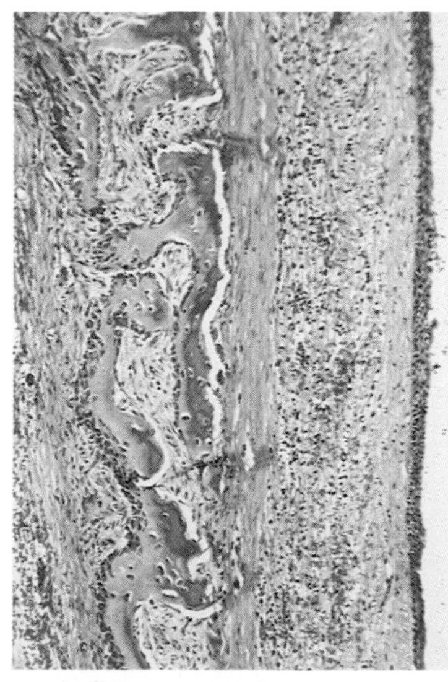

Fig. 52 Complete epithelial, fibrous and bony cyst wall.

Radicular cysts (2)

Microscopy

Clefts

Cholesterol from the breakdown of blood cells is frequently seen in cysts as needle-shaped clefts. Clefts typically form in the cyst wall but extend into the cyst cavity (Fig. 53, Fig. 58, p. 30). Clefts are surrounded by giant cells whose cytoplasm becomes stretched and attenuated, but the clusters of nuclei may be seen near one end (Fig. 54).

Aspiration of cyst fluid typically also shows cholesterol as flat, rhomboid, notched crystals (Fig. 55) often with many inflammatory cells.

Microscopy

Hyaline bodies

Hyaline (Rushton) bodies are thin refractile rod-like or hair-pin or other shapes (Fig. 56). Staining is variable. Their nature is unknown. They may be an epithelial product or haematogenous in origin.

Microscopy

Goblet cells

Mucous metaplasia can produce mucin-filled goblet cells in the epithelial lining of radicular cysts but considerably more frequently in dentigerous cysts (see Fig. 59, p. 30).

Behaviour and prognosis

Competent enucleation of radicular cysts is curative. Complications of such treatment are rare. Neglected cysts can become infected or grow until the jaw fractures.

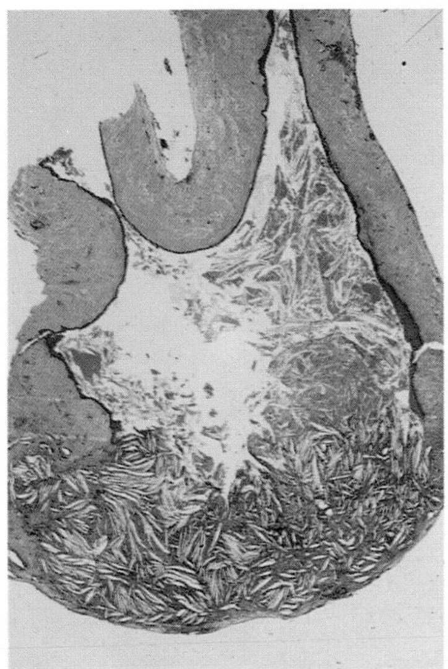

Fig. 53 Cleft formation in the wall of a cyst.

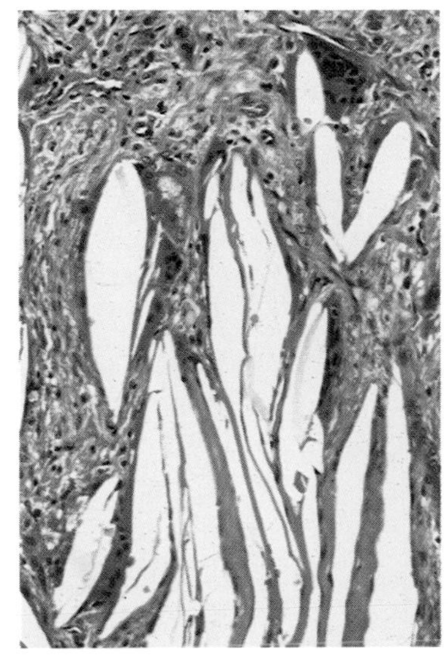

Fig. 54 Clefts in giant cells and deposits of haemosiderin.

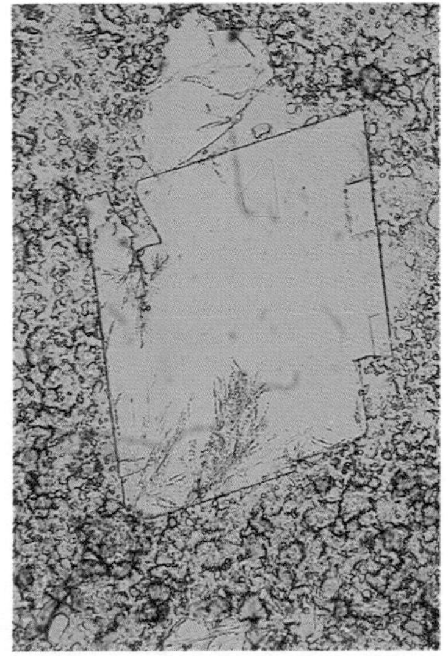

Fig. 55 Cholesterol crystal from cyst fluid.

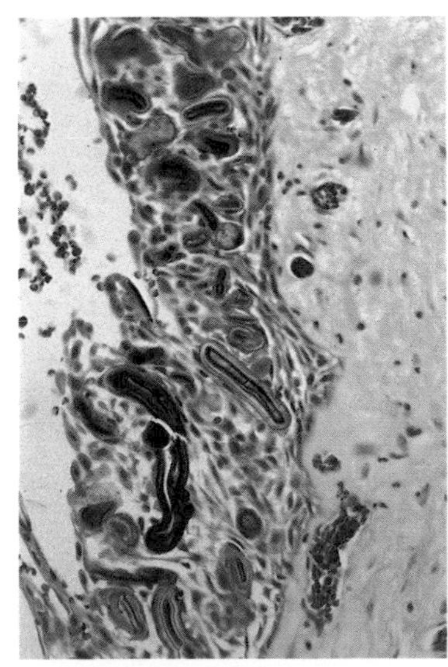

Fig. 56 Hyaline bodies in cyst wall.

Dentigerous cysts

Aetiology

Cystic change in remains of enamel organ after completion of enamel formation. This is a developmental defect of unknown cause.

Incidence

15–18% of jaw cysts. The male:female ratio is more than 2:1.

Microscopy

The cyst wall is attached to the neck of the tooth at or near the amelocemental junction (Figs 57 & 58).

The lining of the cyst (probably originating from external enamel epithelium) typically appears as a thin flat layer of squamous cells without a defined layer of basal cells. The inner enamel epithelium covering the crown of the tooth is usually lost. The fibrous wall is typically without inflammatory infiltrate, unless secondarily infected. Mucous cells are relatively common (Fig. 59).

Behaviour and prognosis

Competent enucleation of dentigerous cysts with extraction of the contained tooth is curative. Occasionally, if space is available, the cyst can be marsupialized and the tooth persuaded to erupt into a functional position.

Eruption cysts

An eruption cyst is, strictly, a soft tissue cyst in the gingiva overlying an unerupted tooth. It is probably a superficial dentigerous cyst.

Microscopy

Thin fibrous wall with thin squamous epithelial lining deeply and oral mucosal epithelium superficially (Fig. 60). There is variable inflammatory infiltrate in the wall.

Eruption cysts usually rupture spontaneously.

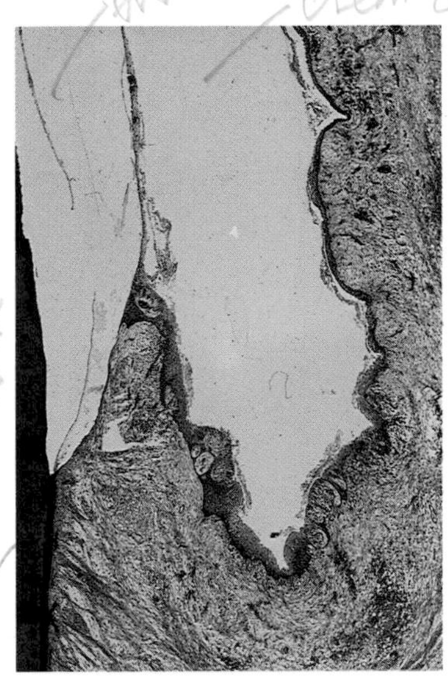

Fig. 57 Dentigerous cyst with enamel epithelium between enamel space (left) and cyst (right).

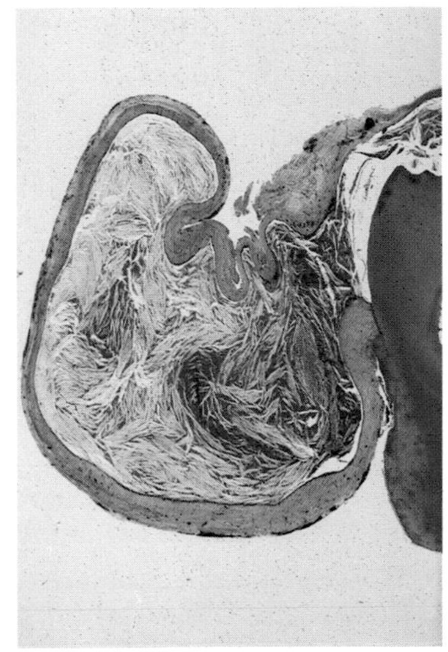

Fig. 58 Dentigerous cyst showing attachment at neck of tooth.

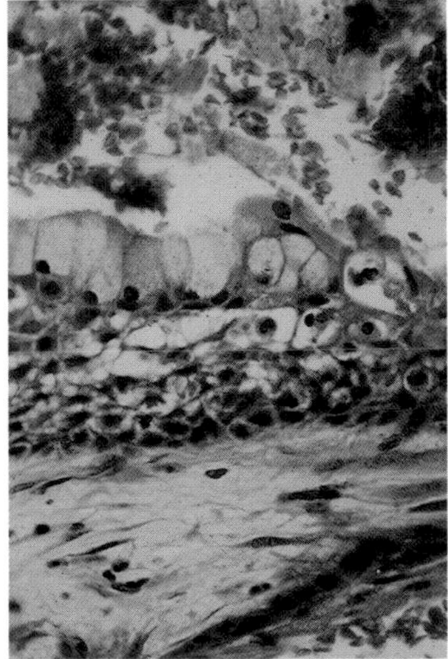

Fig. 59 Goblet cells in dentigerous cyst lining.

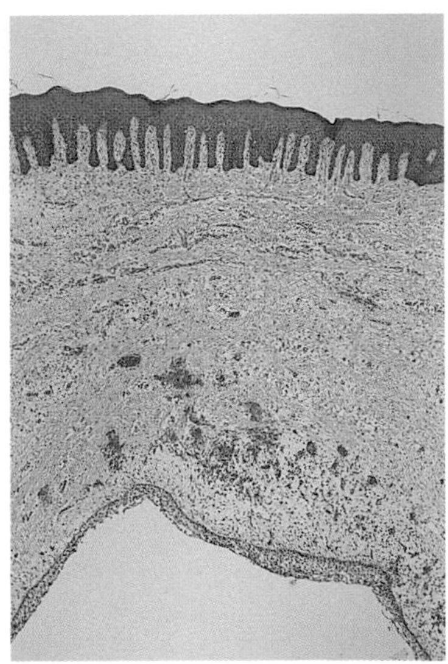

Fig. 60 Eruption cyst. Mucosal epithelium covers the roof of the cyst.

Odontogenic keratocyst

Aetiology

Unknown. Probably originates from primordial odontogenic epithelium (any part of dental lamina or remnants thereof) or enamel organ before the start of amelogenesis. A tooth is sometimes missing.

Incidence

About 10% of odontogenic cysts. The male to female ratio is about 1.5:1. They form most frequently in young adults or at age 50–60; possibly then as a result of slow growth and late detection.

Radiography

About 75% in body or ramus of mandible. Typically, expansive growth into cancellous bone forms an extensive multilocular area of radiolucency with little expansion of bone.

Microscopy

Characteristic lining of epithelium of even thickness, 5–8 cells thick, and flat basement membrane. There is usually a tall, palisaded basal cell layer and thin eosinophilic layer of parakeratin (Fig. 61).

Orthokeratinization is seen in a minority (about 30%), occasionally with keratin forming semisolid cyst contents (Fig. 62).

Parakeratinized cysts. The epithelium is typically much folded and tends to separate from the fibrous wall (Fig. 63). Daughter cysts are occasionally seen in the cyst wall and may account for some recurrences (see Fig. 65, p. 34). An inflammatory infiltrate is typically absent but infection and inflammation cause the lining to resemble that of a radicular cyst (Fig. 64).

Behaviour and prognosis

Unlike the common odontogenic cysts, keratocysts—particularly the parakeratinized type—have a strong tendency to recur after treatment, sometimes decades later. Recurrence rates of up to 60% have been recorded in the past. The extensive, infiltrative pattern of growth and the weak attachment of the epithelium to the cyst wall, allowing fragments to be left behind, probably contribute.

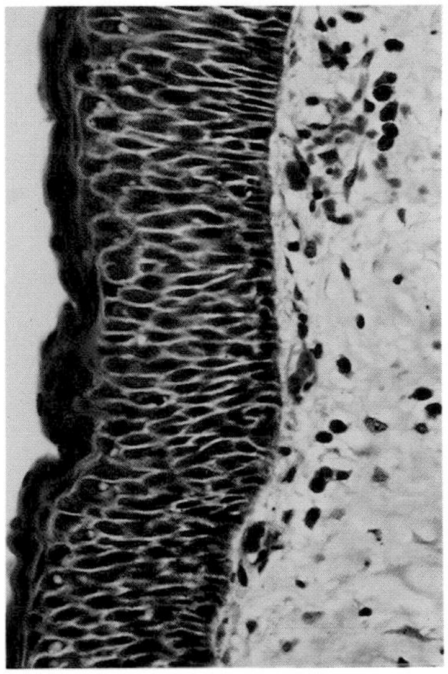

Fig. 61 Typical parakeratinized keratocyst lining.

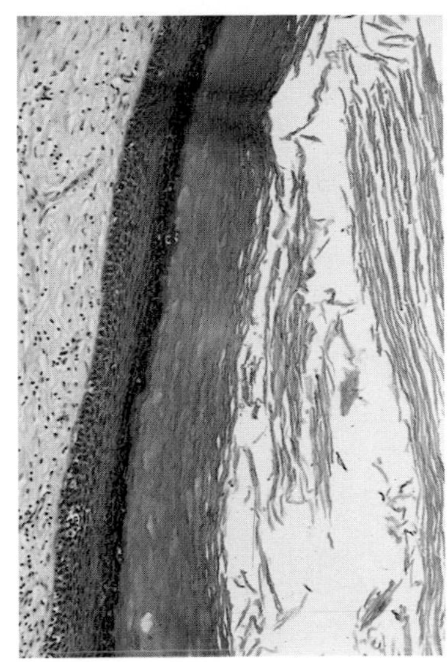

Fig. 62 Keratocyst with orthokeratinization.

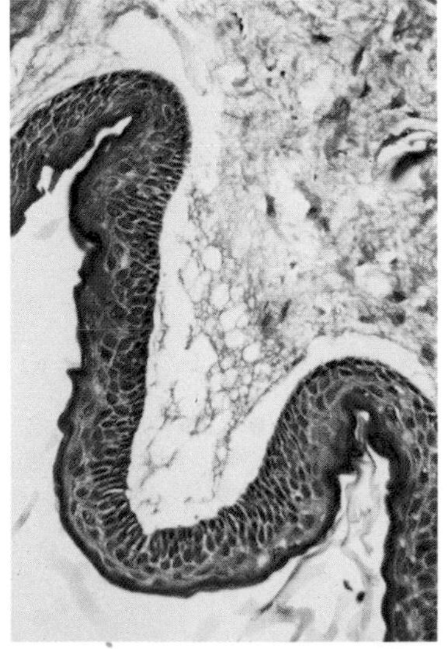

Fig. 63 Keratocyst, parakeratinized type, showing weak attachment to cyst wall.

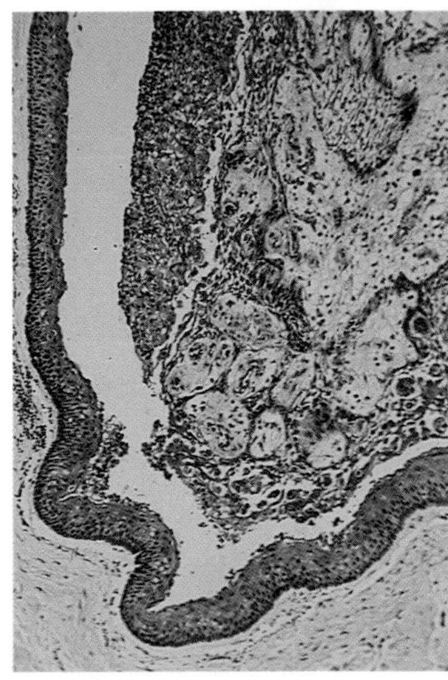

Fig. 64 Keratocyst showing loss of typical structure as a result of inflammation.

Nasopalatine duct (incisive canal) cyst

Aetiology

Proliferation of epithelial remnants of lining of nasopalatine duct.

Microscopy

Midline cyst of anterior maxilla with lining of squamous and/or ciliated columnar epithelium (Fig. 66). Characteristically, a neurovascular bundle (also from incisive canal) (Fig. 67) and sometimes salivary acini may be found in the cyst wall.

Nasolabial cyst

Aetiology

Unknown. This is an exceedingly rare soft tissue cyst external to the alveolar ridge beneath the ala nasi. It probably arises from remnants of the lower end of the nasolacrimal duct. A nasolabial cyst may be seen at almost any age but the peak incidence is at 40–50 years.

Microscopy

The lining classically (but often not) is of non-ciliated columnar epithelium but may be squamous or ciliated with a fibrous wall (Fig. 68).

Behaviour and prognosis

Enucleation is effective.

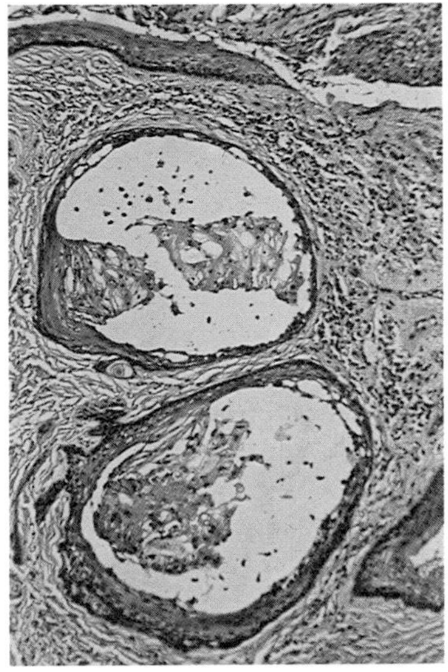

Fig. 65 Daughter cysts in keratocyst wall.

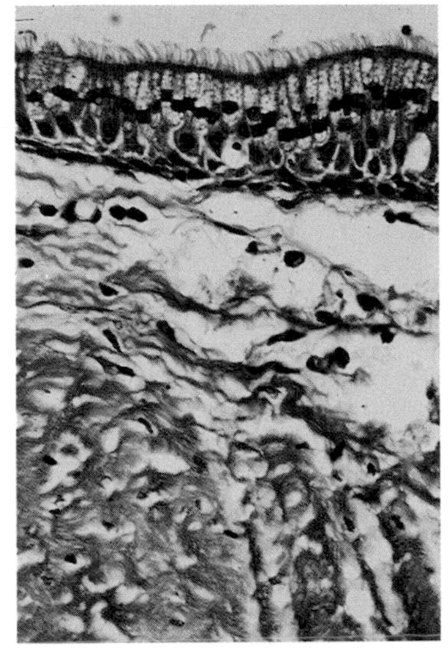

Fig. 66 Ciliated epithelium lining nasopalatine cyst.

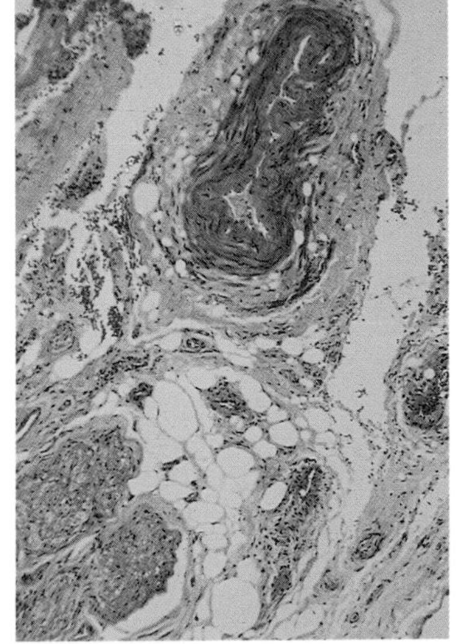

Fig. 67 Neurovascular bundle in nasopalatine cyst wall.

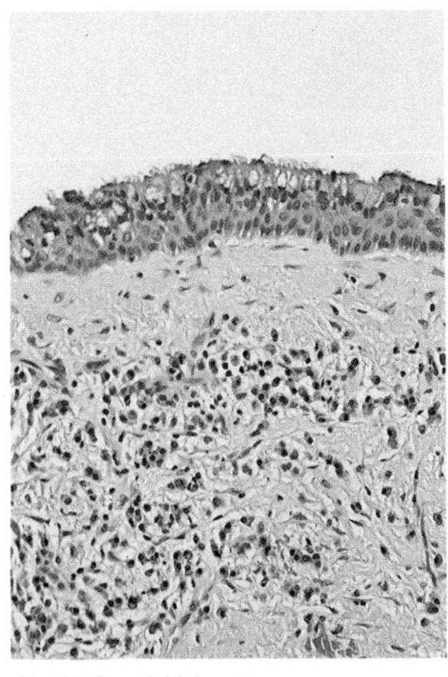

Fig. 68 Nasolabial cyst.

Cystic odontogenic tumours

The main examples are the *unicystic ameloblastoma* (see p. 44) and the *calcifying odontogenic (ghost cell) cyst*.

Microscopy

Cystic ameloblastoma

Extensive cystic change (Fig. 69) can overgrow the tumour. The lining becomes flattened and may be indistinguishable in part from that of a simple cyst. Elsewhere, ameloblastoma cells are more obvious in the cyst lining and a typical tumour forms mural thickening.

Calcifying odontogenic (ghost cell) cyst

Incidence

Rare. Any age can be affected but the lesion is most often detected in the second decade.

Microscopy

Fibrous wall with lining predominantly of squamous epithelium but the basal layer cells may be columnar and ameloblast-like. Abnormal keratinization of spinous cells produces ghost cells consisting of distended eosinophilic epithelial cells either anuclear or occasionally containing nuclear remnants (Figs 70–72). Patchy calcification may develop in them. Associated or induced odontogenic tumours or hamartomas are not infrequent, developing in the adjacent fibrous wall.

Behaviour and prognosis

Curettage is usually adequate. Recurrences are uncommon but respond to more extensive curettage or excision. Spontaneous resolution has occasionally been reported.

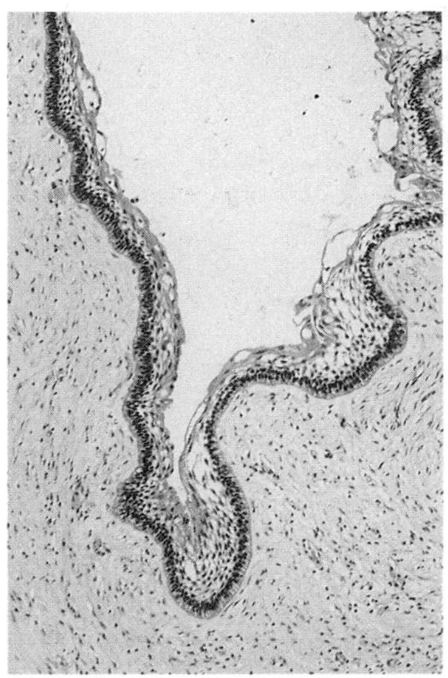

Fig. 69 Cyst in ameloblastoma.

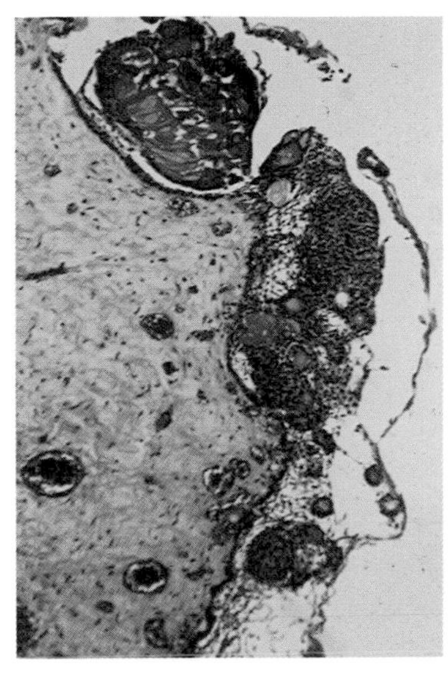

Fig. 70 Calcifying odontogenic cyst with ghost cells.

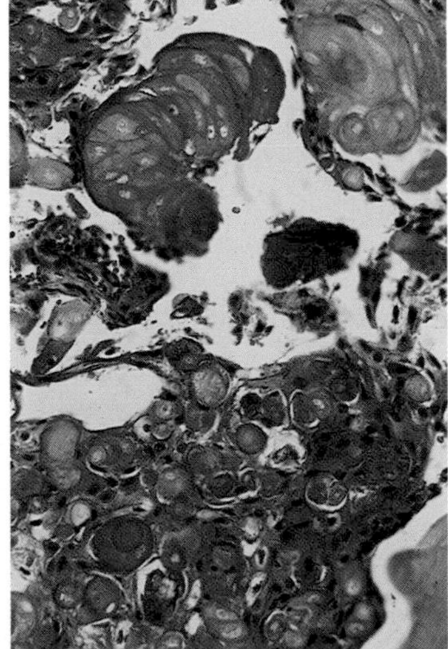

Fig. 71 Calcifying odontogenic cyst with ghost cells.

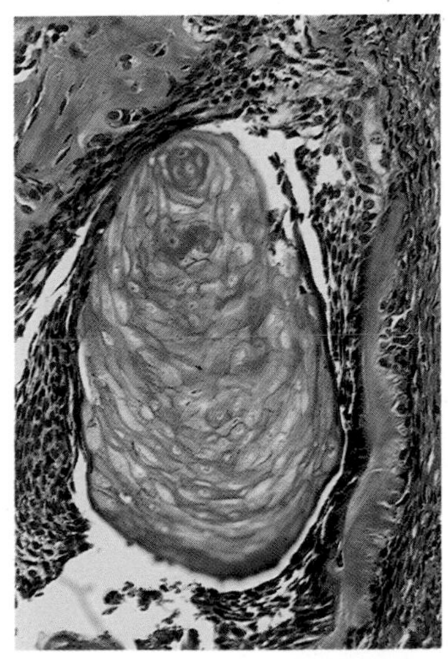

Fig. 72 Calcifying odontogenic cyst with ghost cells.

Cysts without epithelial lining (non-odontogenic pseudocysts)

Solitary bone cyst

Incidence and aetiology

Rare, but with peak age incidence in the second decade. The aetiology is speculative. Traditionally thought to be traumatic (earlier terms: haemorrhagic or traumatic bone cyst), but no supporting evidence.

Almost invariably in mandible. The cavity and radiolucency extend through cancellous bone and arch up between the roots of teeth but rarely expand the bone.

Microscopy

The cyst may contain serosanguinous fluid or be empty except for air. The wall is usually rough, bare bone, sometimes with traces of connective tissue as incomplete lining (Fig. 73), often with evidence of small haemorrhages.

Prognosis

Unlike true cysts, solitary bone cysts probably heal spontaneously. The cavity should be opened only to confirm the diagnosis. The resulting bleeding into the cavity causes it to heal, i.e. these cysts are not *caused* by bleeding into the bone.

Aneurysmal bone cyst

Aetiology

Speculative. Possibly this is a developmental vascular defect or a result of bleeding into, or vascularization of, a pre-existing lesion such as a giant cell granuloma.

Pathology

Grossly, the cyst resembles a blood-filled sponge. Microscopically, it consists of blood-filled spaces lined by flattened cells and separated by highly vascular connective tissue septa and similar solid areas often with many giant cells (Figs 74 & 75). Sometimes the solid areas may calcify and resemble ossifying fibroma.

Prognosis

Excision is usually curative.

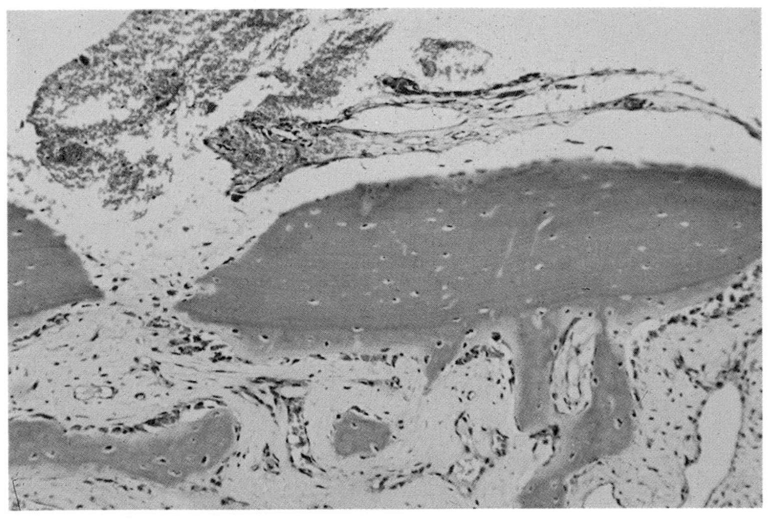

Fig. 73 Solitary bone cyst: scanty, incomplete lining (above).

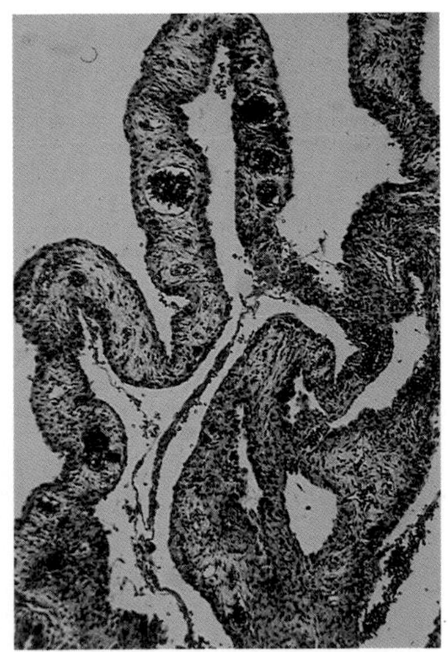

Fig. 74 Aneurysmal bone cyst.

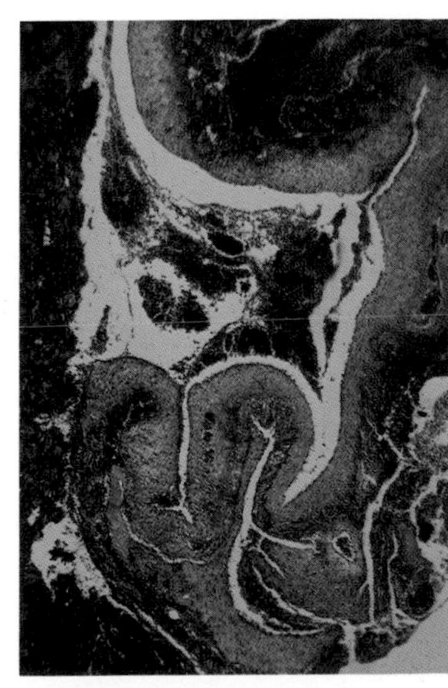

Fig. 75 Aneurysmal bone cyst.

8 / Odontogenic tumours

Ameloblastoma (1)

Most common neoplasm of jaws. Mainly affects males aged over 40 years, with about 80% of tumours in the ramus or posterior body of the mandible. Typically appears as a multilocular cyst on a radiograph. Occasionally monolocular, can mimic a radicular or dentigerous cyst. Slow growing and locally invasive but does not metastasize.

Microscopy

Several subtypes are recognized.

Follicular type: islands or trabeculae of loose angular cells, resembling stellate reticulum, surrounded by a single layer of tall, columnar, ameloblast-like cells with nuclei at the opposite pole to the basement membrane (Figs 76–78). Cyst formation varies from microcysts within a solid tumour to a predominantly cystic tumour (see Fig. 83, p. 44). Cysts develop either within epithelial islands (Figs 76 & 77) or from cystic degeneration of connective tissue stroma—only the ghosts of blood vessels may remain (Fig. 79). In *cystic ameloblastoma*, the lining is often flattened, resembling a non-neoplastic cyst (see Fig. 83, p. 44).

Plexiform type: thin trabeculae of epithelial cells in connective tissue stroma (see Fig. 80, p. 42).

Acanthomatous type: squamous metaplasia of central core of epithelium, but otherwise resembles the more common follicular type (Fig. 81, p. 42).

Basal cell type: small, darkly staining cells, predominantly in a trabecular pattern but with little palisading at the periphery. Rare, extraosseous basal cell ameloblastomas have been mistaken for basal cell carcinomas.

Granular cell type: rare, usually resembles the follicular type, but tumour islands contain large eosinophilic granular epithelial cells (see Fig. 84, p. 44). ➡

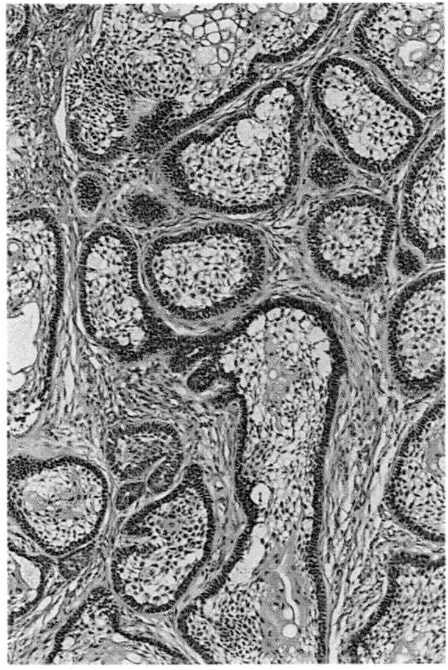

Fig. 76 Ameloblastoma, follicular type.

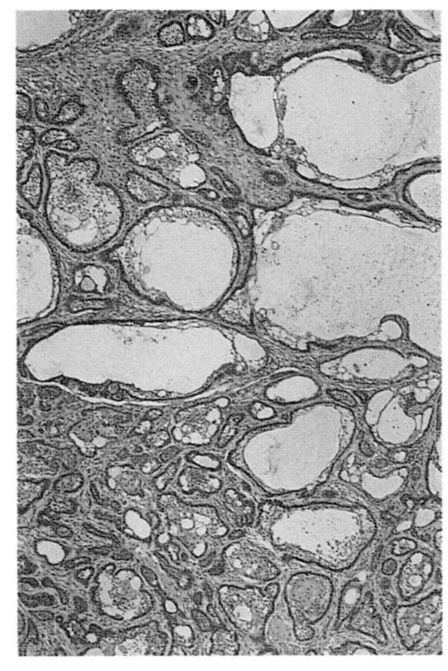

Fig. 77 Ameloblastoma, follicular type. Low power view showing follicles of tumour with central microcyst formation.

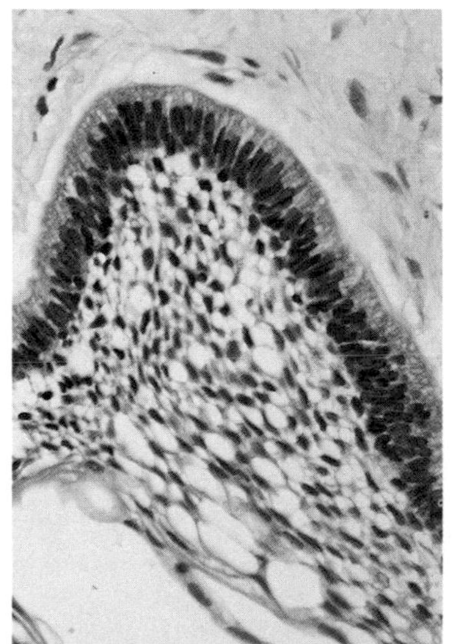

Fig. 78 Ameloblastoma: ameloblast-like cells.

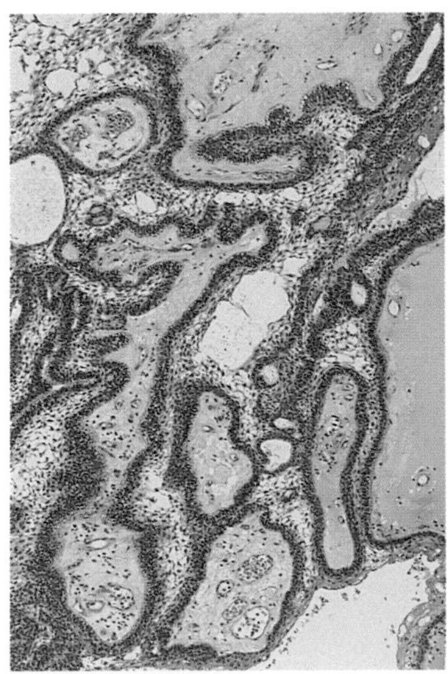

Fig. 79 Ameloblastoma showing stromal and epithelial cysts.

Ameloblastoma (2)

Desmoplastic ameloblastomas are rare. Radiographic appearances include irregular radiolucent areas usually with indistinct borders and containing fine irregular calcifications. Others are mixed radiolucent/radiopaque with indistinct borders.

Microscopically, this variant may be difficult to recognize as an ameloblastoma. Dense collagenous fibrous tissue encloses small, irregular, islands of neoplastic epithelium. There is little or no cyst formation and ameloblast-like cells are typically only present in small foci, surrounding some islands of epithelium. The interior of the epithelial islands consists of densely packed spindle-shaped or polygonal cells with occasional foci of squamous metaplasia centrally. Calcification in the fibrous stroma and occasionally bone formation is seen.

Unicystic ameloblastomas are uncommon. They more frequently affect patients >30 years old; males are affected twice as frequently as females.

Unicystic ameloblastoma is defined as a single cystic cavity which shows ameloblastomatous differentiation in the lining. The unilocular cyst may have a flattened lining but often with typical ameloblastoma cells in the basal layer only in some parts, and no infiltration of the wall by neoplasm. Alternatively there may be intraluminal proliferation without infiltration of the cyst wall. In yet other cases there may be plexiform or follicular ameloblastoma infiltrating the cyst wall. In all these circumstances, the lining of the cystic area becomes flattened and can resemble that of a non-neoplastic cyst. Biopsy of a small part of the cyst wall therefore may be unrepresentative and lead to it being misdiagnosed as a non-neoplastic cyst.

The majority surround a misplaced molar tooth and appear radiographically as dentigerous cysts.

Unicystic ameloblastomas, with no neoplastic infiltration of the cyst wall have a much better prognosis than conventional ameloblastomas. Even when enucleated as cysts, the recurrence rate may be only 10%. However, if there is neoplastic infiltration of the cyst wall, the tumour should be treated as a conventional ameloblastoma. ➡

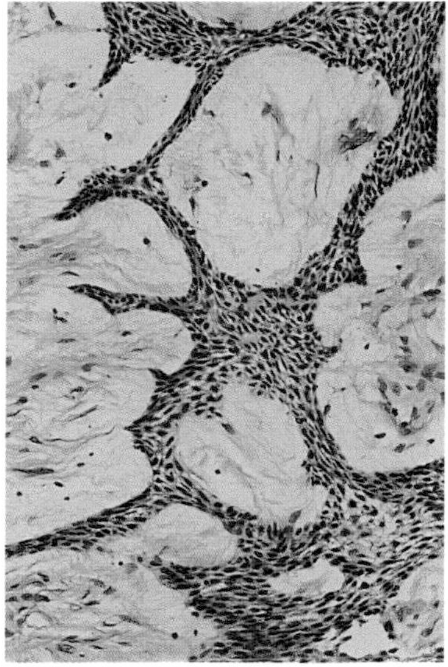

Fig. 80 Ameloblastoma, plexiform type.

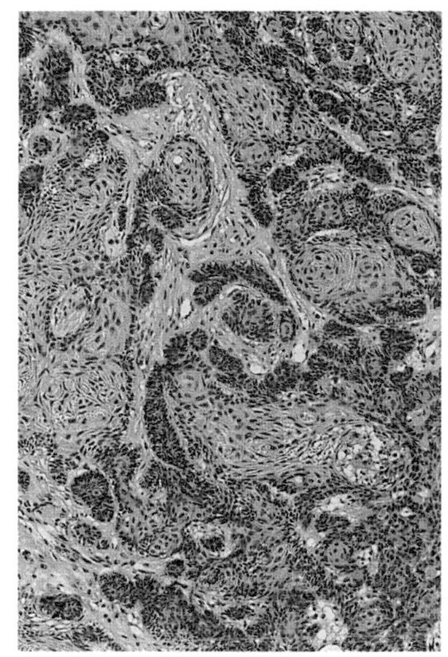

Fig. 81 Ameloblastoma, acanthomatous type. Squamous epithelium forms the bulk of the central cells.

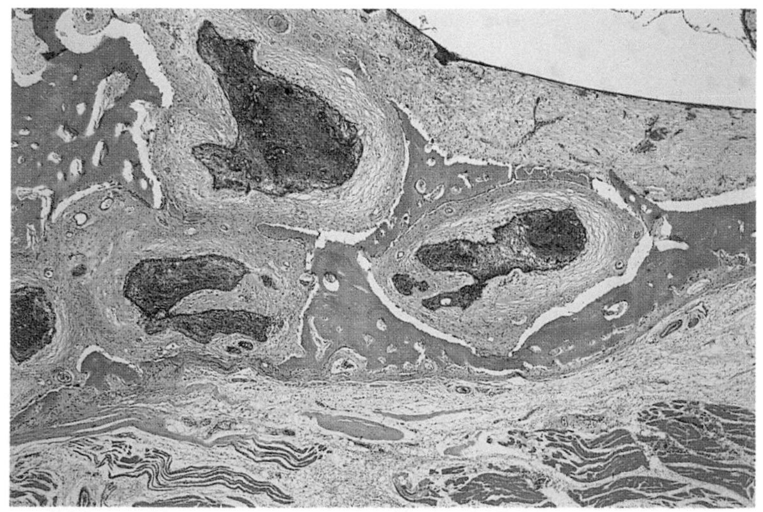

Fig. 82 Ameloblastoma. Finger-like extensions of tumour appear as islands within the mandibular bone.

Ameloblastoma (3)

Maxillary ameloblastomas are particularly dangerous partly because the bones are considerably thinner than those of the mandible and offer weak barriers to spread. Maxillary ameloblastomas tend to form in the posterior segment and to grow upwards to invade the sinonasal passages, pterygomaxillary fossa, orbit, cranium and brain, sometimes fatally.

Prognosis

The histological variants of solid ameloblastomas have not been convincingly shown to affect behaviour and a few have mixed histological patterns. Maxillary ameloblastomas may be more cellular are more frequently plexiform. They certainly have a worse prognosis, probably because of the ease with which the tumour can penetrate the thin maxillary bones to reach the skull base. Ameloblastomas extending into the soft tissues may also be difficult to manage. As mentioned earlier, unicystic ameloblastomas frequently respond to enucleation alone.

Behaviour

Biopsy is essential, particularly for cystic ameloblastomas where a recognizable tumour may be present only as a limited area of mural thickening. Differentiation from non-neoplastic cysts or other radiolucent lesions by radiography alone is unreliable. Ameloblastomas are invasive and recur unless widely excised. The monolocular, unicystic variant may respond to thorough enucleation. Rare maxillary ameloblastomas may present major surgical problems if they invade the cranial cavity. Ameloblastomas spreading into soft tissues (Fig. 83) are also difficult to manage.

Treatment

Ideally, treatment is by complete excision, preferably with up to a 2 cm margin of normal bone. However, spread is mainly through cancellous bone and it is sometimes possible to preserve the lower border of the mandible, if it is tumour-free, to avoid complete resection of the jaw. Bony repair can re-form much of the jaw. Any residual tumour is slow growing and any recurrence should be detectable by regular radiographic follow-up, allowing further limited excision if necessary.

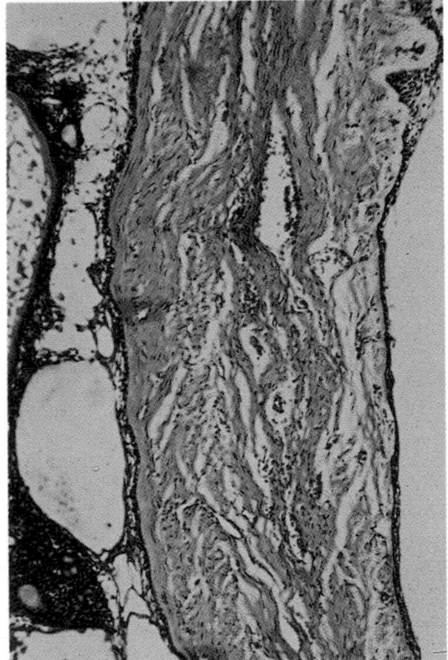

Fig. 83 Cystic ameloblastoma.

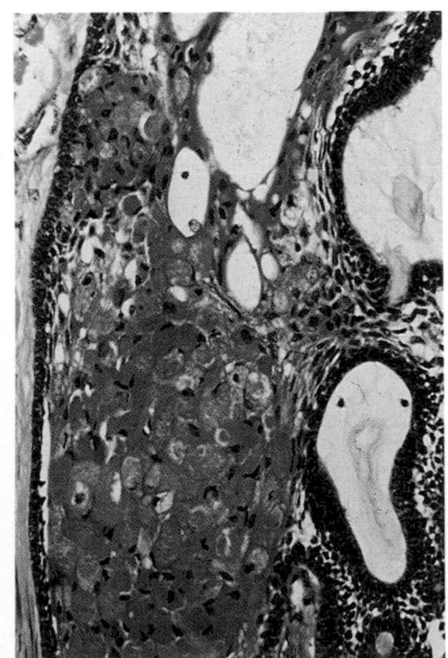

Fig. 84 Ameloblastoma: granular cells.

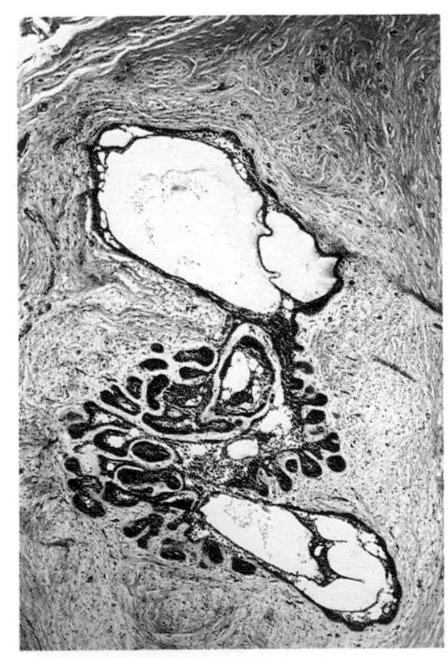

Fig. 85 Soft tissue extension of ameloblastoma.

Calcifying odontogenic (ghost cell) 'cyst'

Solid variant (Fig. 86) of lesion described earlier (p. 35).

Calcifying epithelial odontogenic (Pindborg) tumour (CEOT)

This is a rare but important tumour because of its resemblance to and risk of confusion with poorly differentiated carcinoma. Age and site distribution are similar to that of ameloblastoma.

Radiographic appearances are variable: there may be circumscribed or diffuse radiolucency often with scattered snow-shower opacities. Trabeculation is also variable—multilocular, honeycomb or monolocular appearances may be seen.

Microscopy

Sheets of variable-sized squamous cells, typically with well-defined cell membranes and prominent intercellular bridges (Fig. 87). The nuclei are often pleomorphic, large and hyperchromatic resembling carcinoma (Fig. 88), or smaller and more uniform (Fig. 89). Variations in appearance do not appear to affect behaviour. The connective tissue stroma, unlike carcinomas, lacks an inflammatory infiltrate.

The tumour may also contain calcifications (Fig. 89) and, characteristically, deposits of amyloid-like material (Fig. 88). A few clear cells may be present but the *clear cell odontogenic carcinoma* is a different entity, without amyloid or calcifications, and can metastasize.

Behaviour

Behaviour of CEOT is rather similar to that of ameloblastoma, with slow but invasive growth and a tendency to recur if not fully excised.

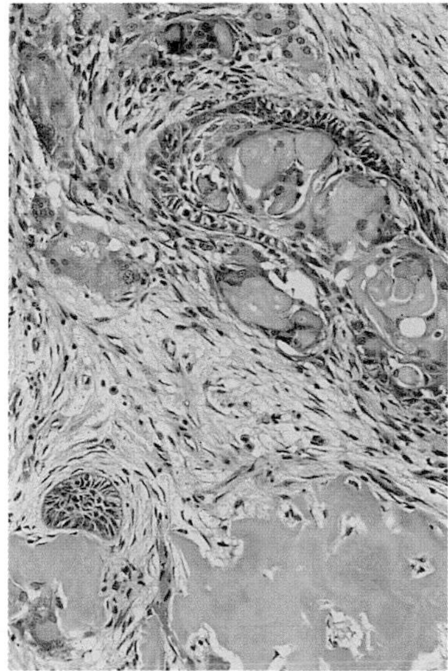

Fig. 86 Calcifying odontogenic (ghost cell) cyst: solid type showing ameloblast-like cells.

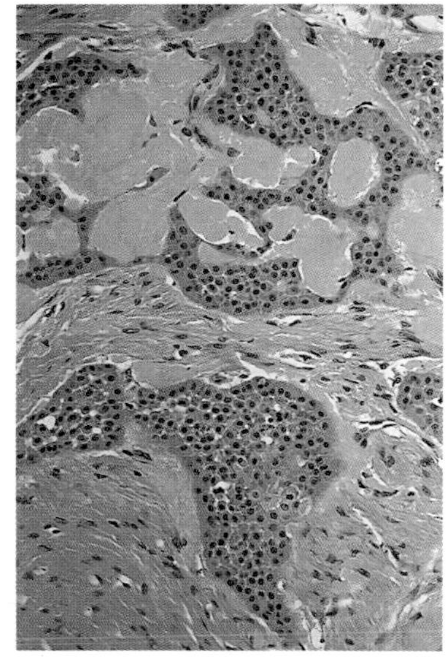

Fig. 87 Calcifying epithelial odontogenic tumour. Neoplastic epithelium with large hyperchromatic nuclei surrounds pinkish amyloid-like material.

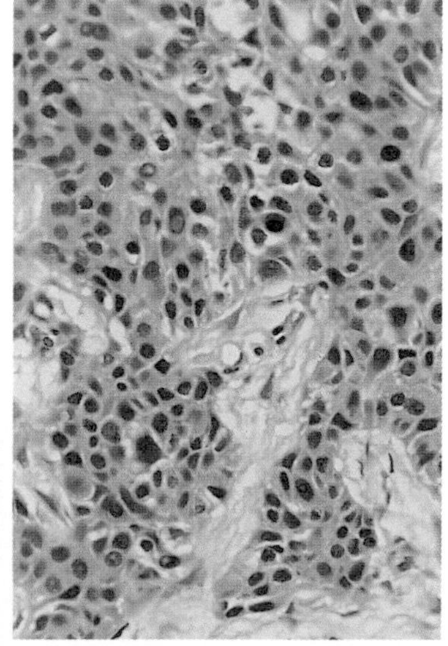

Fig. 88 CEOT. Conspicuous pleomorphism and hyperchromatism of the epithelial nuclei.

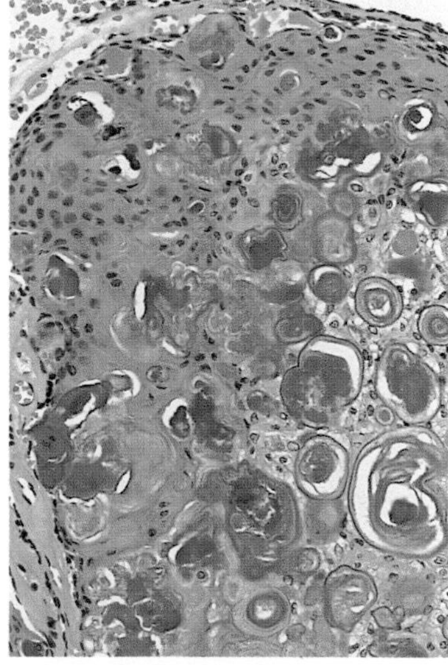

Fig. 89 CEOT. Calcifications.

Adenomatoid odontogenic tumour

Mainly found in teens or twenties and has a higher incidence in women than in men. The anterior maxilla is usually affected.

The tumour surrounds, or is contiguous with, a tooth, producing a radiographic appearance similar to that of a radicular or dentigerous cyst.

Microscopy

Consists of whorls or sheets of small, dark epithelial cells (Fig. 90), frequently with amorphous or crystalline calcifications and microcysts (resembling ducts in cross-section) lined by ameloblast-like columnar epithelium (Fig. 91). There is a fibrous capsule.

Prognosis

The tumour is readily enucleated without risk of recurrence.

Melanotic neuroectodermal tumour of infancy (progonoma)

This is a rare tumour that is not odontogenic but originates from the neural crest. It is usually detected as a ragged area of radiolucency in the maxilla at about 3 months; the mandible or other sites are rarely affected.

Microscopy

Consists of a connective tissue stroma containing foci of pigmented (melanin-containing) cells (Fig. 92) with pale nuclei, surrounding small spaces or clefts, together with groups of non-pigmented cells, alone or surrounded by pigment cells (Fig. 93).

Behaviour

Variable rate of growth, but most appear to be benign and with rare exceptions do not recur after excision.

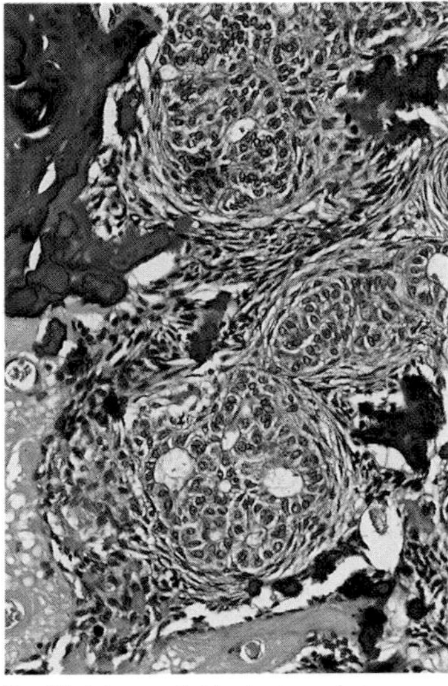

Fig. 90 Adenomatoid odontogenic tumour.

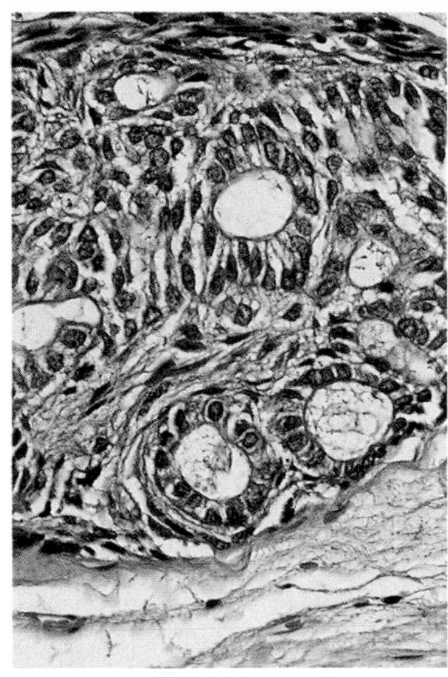

Fig. 91 Adenomatoid odontogenic tumour: microcysts and ameloblast-like cells.

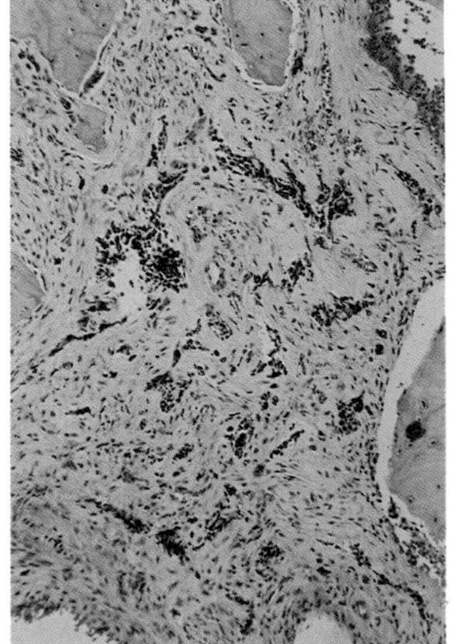

Fig. 92 Melanotic neuroectodermal tumour.

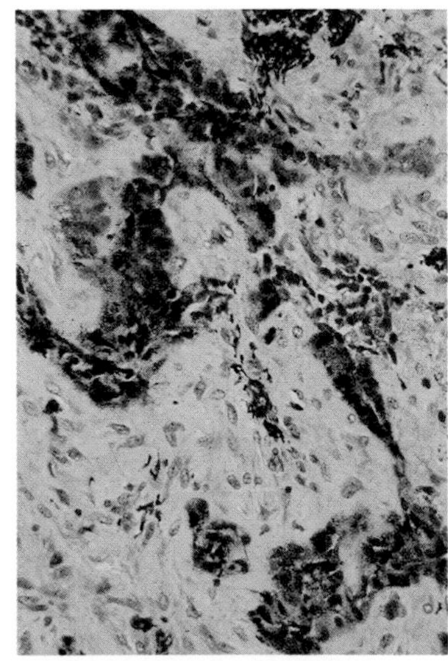

Fig. 93 Melanotic neuroectodermal tumour: pigment cells. (High power.)

Squamous odontogenic tumour

Rare tumour consisting of multiple islands of well-differentiated squamous cells in connective tissue stroma (Figs 94 & 95). It has a wide age distribution and no apparent sex or site predilection.

Microscopy

This appears to be a tumour of the periodontal ligament epithelium and can mimic intrabony periodontal pocketing radiographically.

Behaviour and prognosis

This tumour is benign, and invasion of adjacent structures by maxillary lesions has rarely been reported. Curettage or conservative resection and extraction of any teeth involved is usually effective.

Ameloblastic fibroma

Exceedingly rare and typically affects children and teenagers. It forms a slow-growing, painless swelling with a cyst-like area of radiolucency.

Microscopy

Processes of epithelium resembling ameloblasts surround cells resembling stellate reticulum (Figs 96 & 97). The stroma resembles dentine papilla (Fig. 97). This is thought to be a true mixed tumour and is sometimes associated with a developing composite odontoma.

Prognosis

The tumour is readily enucleated but may recur. Sarcomatous change of the fibrous component is a rare complication.

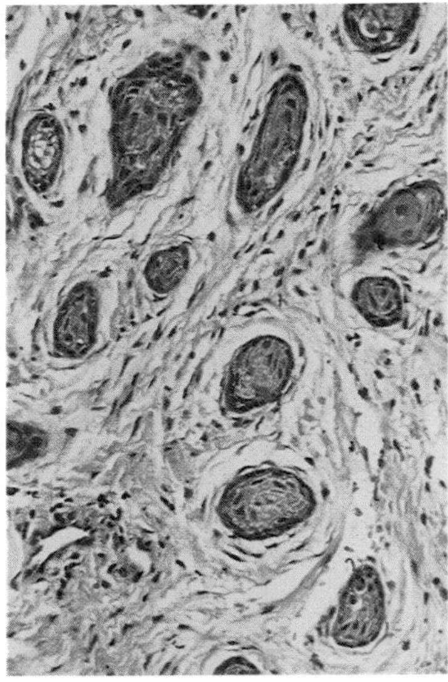

Fig. 94 Squamous odontogenic tumour.

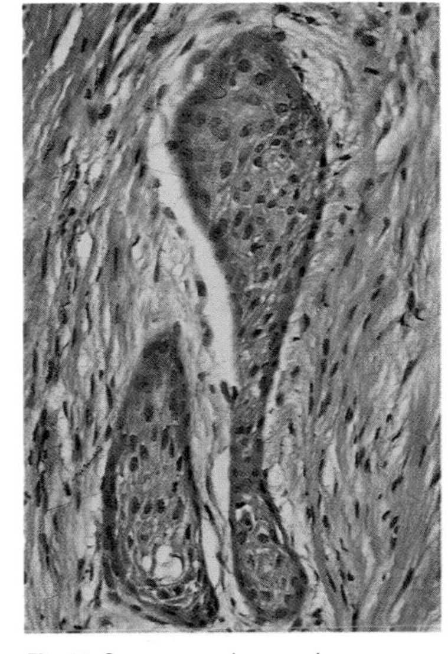

Fig. 95 Squamous odontogenic tumour. (High power.)

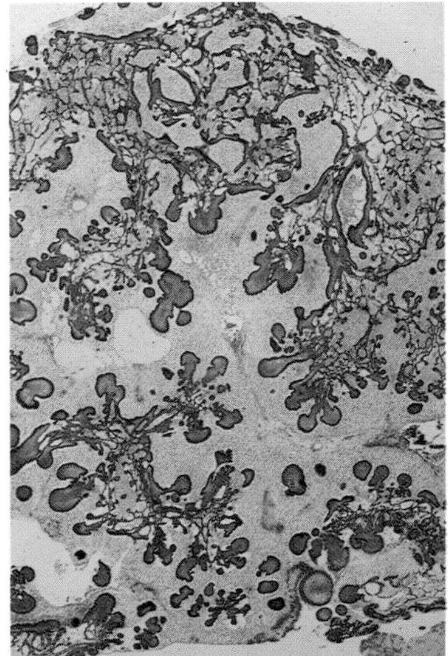

Fig. 96 Ameloblastic fibroma.

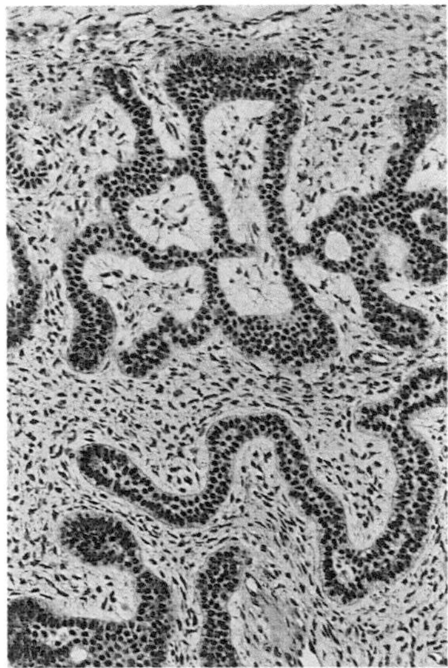

Fig. 97 Ameloblastic fibroma. Darkly staining processes of epithelium are surrounded by highly cellular mesenchyme.

Odontogenic myxoma

Probably arises from the mesenchymal component of tooth germ. Usually detected in the second or third decade, slightly more frequently in the mandible, as a cyst-like or soap bubble area of radiolucency with expansion of bone (Fig. 98).

Microscopy

Loose, mucoid fibrillary tissue contains spindle or stellate cells with long, delicate, intertwining processes (Fig. 99) and, rarely, rests of odontogenic epithelium scattered throughout the tumour. Sometimes there is extensive bone invasion.

Treatment and prognosis

Although benign, this tumour is difficult to remove completely and wide excision is necessary. However, the tumour can persist for years or decades afterwards, though without necessarily causing symptoms.

Odontomas

These are malformations of developing dental tissues (hamartomas). Occasionally, an odontoma is associated with a tumour such as ameloblastic fibroma.

Compound type: multiple small tooth-like structures (denticles) within fibrous follicles (Fig. 100).

Complex type: completely irregular mass of dental tissues (Fig. 101). It may have a cauliflower form with dental tissues surrounding a much branched pulp chamber. Though lacking any morphological resemblance to a tooth, complex odontomas have the individual dental tissues in normal relation to one another. Growth ceases when calcification is complete and the mass tends to erupt and frequently then becomes infected.

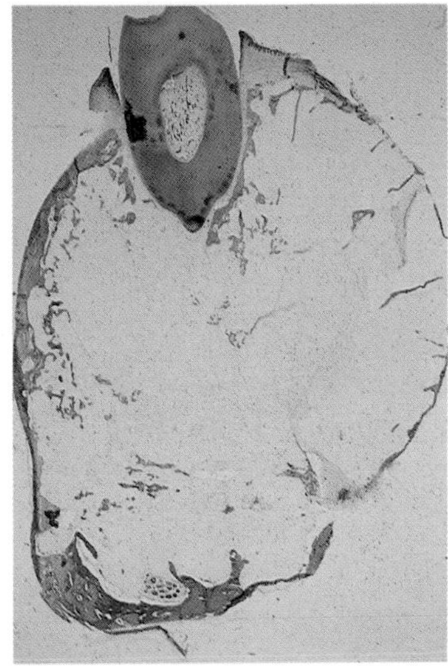

Fig. 98 Odontogenic myxoma.

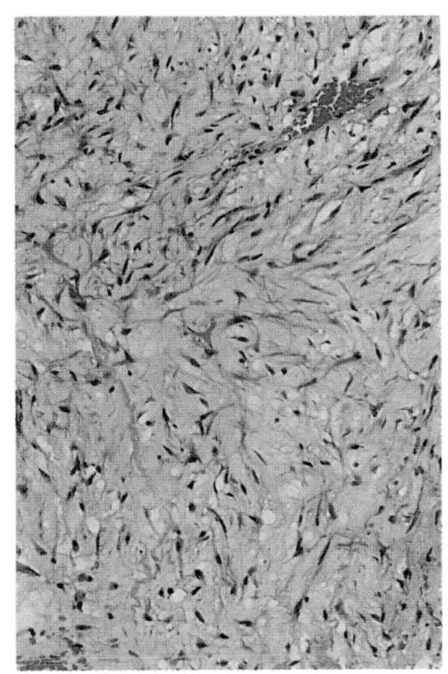

Fig. 99 Myxoma: a cellular example.

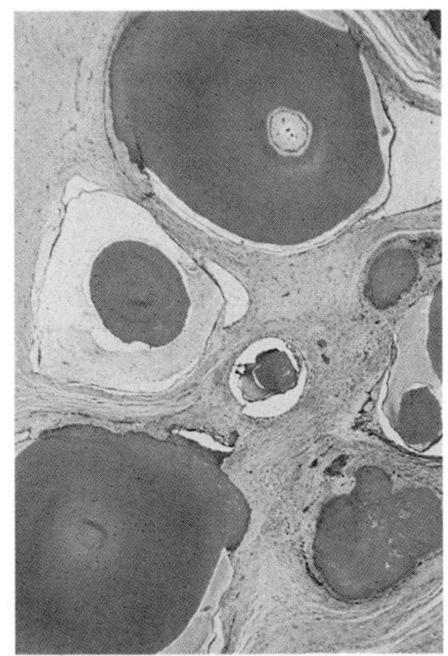

Fig. 100 Compound odontoma.

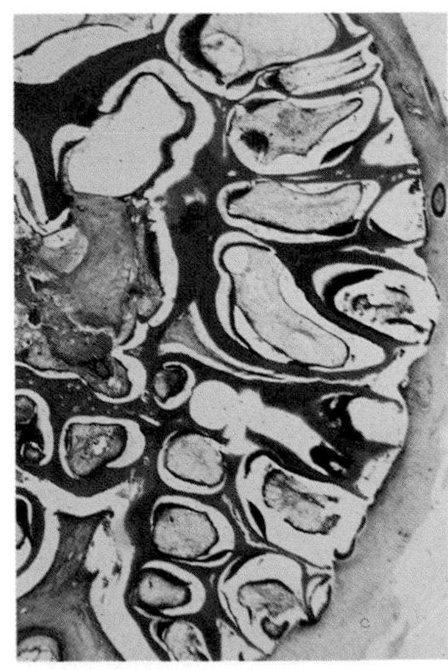

Fig. 101 Complex odontoma.

Cementoblastomas and cemental dysplasias

Cementoblastoma

The tumour usually affects males under 25 years. It appears as a radiopaque apical mass with radiolucent margin, usually in the molar region.

Microscopy

A rounded or irregular mass of cementum can be seen on the root of the tooth (Figs 102 & 103). The cementum is in a pagetoid ('mosaic') pattern with many cementoblasts (Fig. 104), a peripheral zone of pericementum and a zone of uncalcified cement matrix (precementum) and fibrous pericementum.

Behaviour and prognosis

Cementoblastomas are benign but have a potential for continued growth. However, if the related tooth is extracted and the mass completely enucleated, recurrence is rare. If incompletely removed, the mass will continue to grow.

Cemento-ossifying fibroma

No useful distinction can be made between cementifying and ossifying fibromas. Calcifications consist of many cementicle-like ossifications or trabeculae of bone or, frequently, both. Typically found in the mid-30s ages, women being twice as frequently affected. The mandible is the usual site.

Radiographically, cemento-ossifying fibromas have well-defined margins and are radiolucent with varying degrees of calcification. Calcifications tend to be concentrated centrally. Some specimens appear largely radiopaque with a narrow radiolucent rim.

Microscopy

A well-defined capsule surrounds connective tissue of variable cellularity, containing calcifications which also vary widely in type. Calcifications include trabeculae of woven bone, thicker trabeculae of lamellar bone as well as dystrophic calcifications. Minute, rounded cementicle-like, acellular calcifications gradually grow, fuse, and ultimately form a dense mass (Figs 105–107).

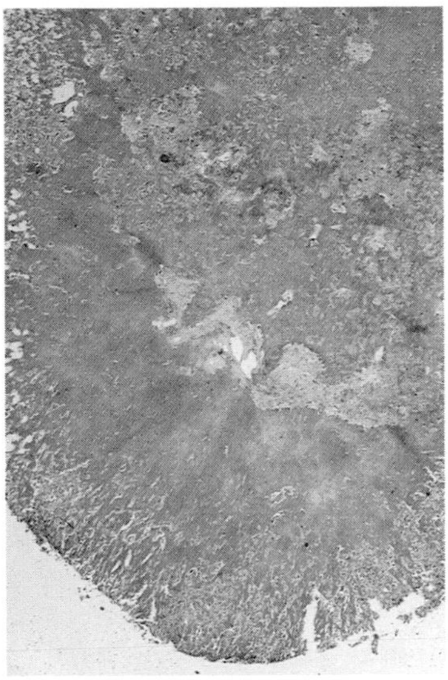

Fig. 102 Cementoblastoma (periphery).

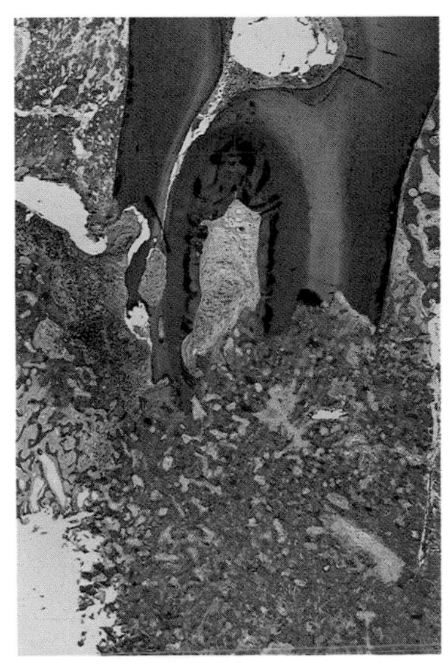

Fig. 103 Cementoblastoma: resorption of related tooth.

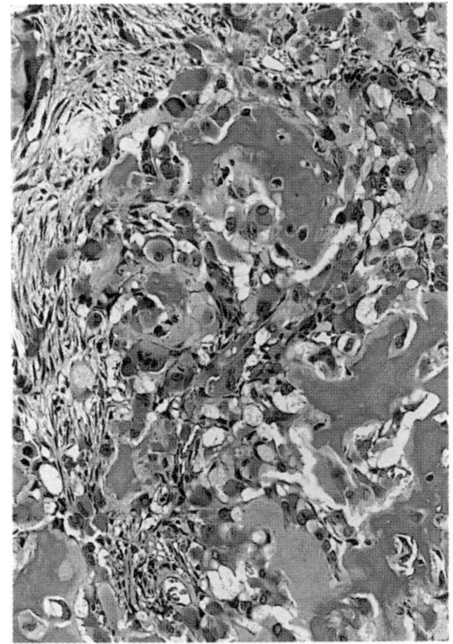

Fig. 104 Cementoblastoma. Cementum-like tissue with many cementoblasts and cementoclasts.

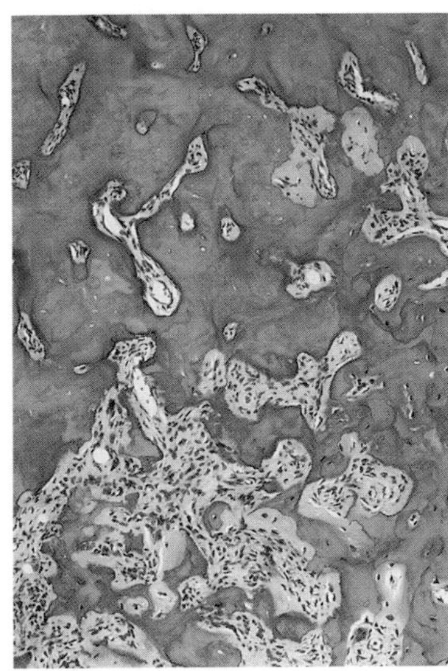

Fig. 105 Cemento-ossifying fibroma.

Behaviour and prognosis

Cemento-ossifying fibromas can be readily enucleated. Rarely, large cementoblastomas which have distorted the jaw require local resection and bone grafting. However if an associated tooth is extracted, a densely calcified cemento-ossifying fibroma can become a focus for chronic osteomyelitis. If this happens, wide excision becomes necessary.

Cemento-osseous dysplasias

Cemento-osseous dysplasias comprise *florid, focal* and *periapical* types. They are of periodontal ligament origin. They predominantly affect women, usually middle-aged, and, overall, blacks are more frequently affected. The mandible is most frequently involved but florid cemento-osseous dysplasia can occupy all four quadrants.

Cemento-osseous dysplasias are typically asymptomatic and appear radiographically as moderately well-defined, mottled radiolucent/opaque or more sclerotic areas of an extent indicated by their names. Periapical cemento-osseous dysplasia may mimic a periapical granuloma in its early stages. The florid type, which appears as irregular or lobulated masses without radiolucent borders interspersed with ill-defined radiolucent/radiopaque areas, may be mistaken for chronic sclerosing osteomyelitis.

Microscopy

The appearances resemble those of cemento-ossifying fibroma. In the early stages, cellular fibrous tissue contains foci of cementum-like tissue which grows and fuses to form a solid, bone-like mass and sometimes, scattered foci of giant cells (Figs 108–109).

Prognosis

Cemento-osseous dysplasias, once fully calcified, appear to have no potential for further growth. The main consideration is to distinguish early lesions from inflammatory disease by dental investigation. Surgical interference, particularly with florid lesions, should be avoided as it can lead to chronic osteomyelitis.

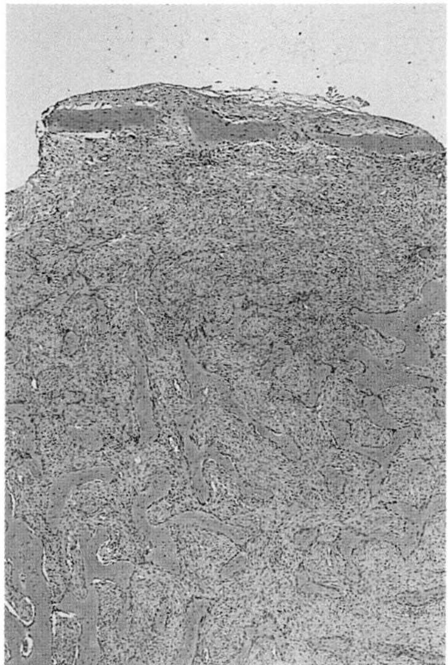

Fig. 106 Cemento-ossifying fibroma. Fine bone trabeculae surrounded by cellular fibrous tissue.

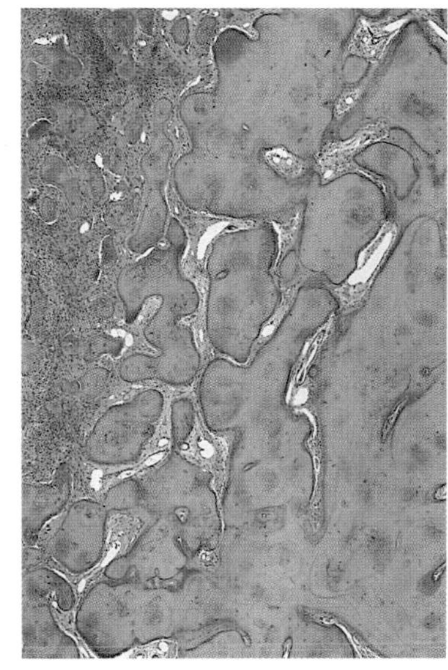

Fig. 107 Cemento-ossifying fibroma. Nodules of cementum-like tissue have fused into large masses.

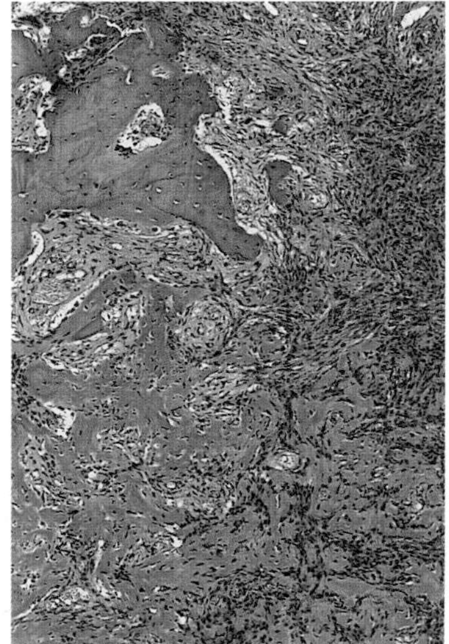

Fig. 108 Florid cemento-osseous dysplasia. Cellular fibrous tissue containing bony and cementum-like tissue.

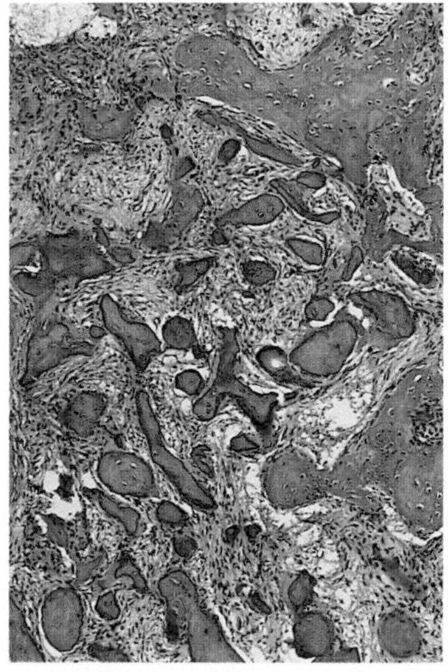

Fig. 109 Florid cemento-osseous dysplasia. Another area also shows cellular fibrous tissue containing bony and cementum-like calcifications.

9 / Nonodontogenic tumours of bone

Chondroma

One of the rarest jaw tumours. It consists of hyaline cartilage containing small chondrocytes in characteristic lacunae. Chondroma is difficult to distinguish from low grade chondrosarcoma.

Osteochondroma (cartilage-capped osteoma)

This is a bony overgrowth with a cartilaginous cap. 95% of cases arise from the coronoid or condylar process.

Microscopy

Hyaline cartilage, often with regularly aligned cells and resembling an epiphysis, overlies slowly proliferating bone, usually cancellous in type (Fig. 110). In time, the mass becomes predominantly bony with a thinning cartilage cap.

Osteoma

May be endosteal or more often periosteal but then it is often difficult to distinguish from an exostosis.

Microscopy

Compact osteoma: lamellae of dense compact bone with relatively few osteocytes (Fig. 111).

Cancellous osteoma: widely spaced bony trabeculae with cortex of lamellated bone (Fig. 112).

Prognosis

Osteochondromas and osteomas are benign and excision is effective.

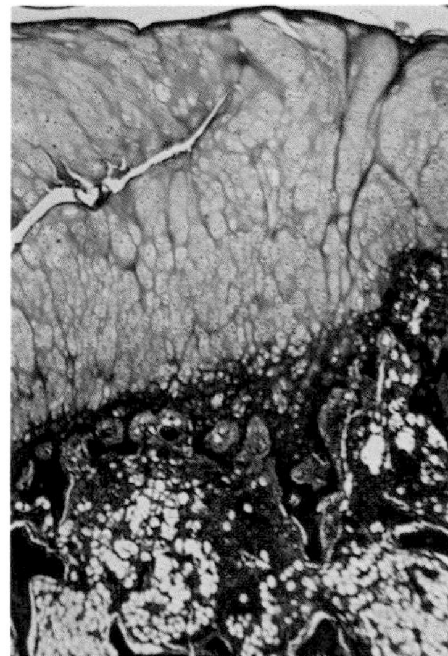

Fig. 110 Osteochondroma.

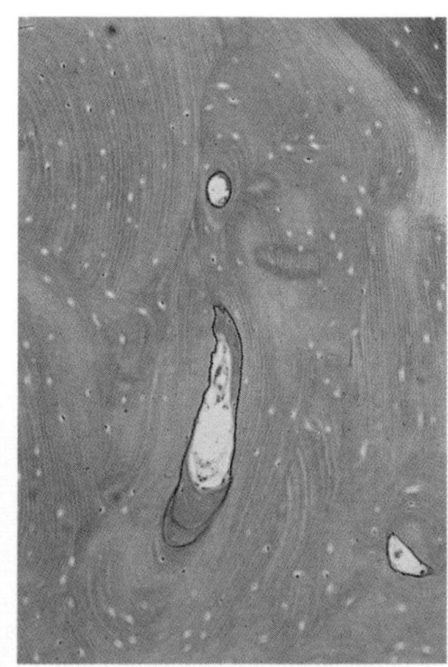

Fig. 111 Compact osteoma.

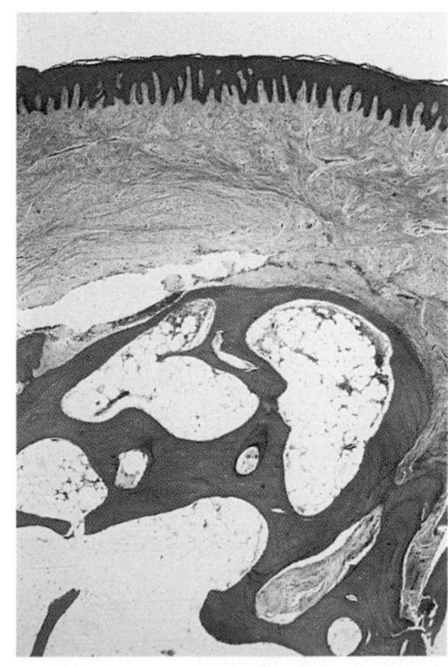

Fig. 112 Cancellous osteoma.

Osteosarcoma

The most common *primary* tumour of bone. It is a rare complication of radiotherapy or Paget's disease of the axial skeleton.

Osteosarcoma usually affects young persons, particularly males.

Radiography

Radiographic features are highly variable corresponding with the variable histopathology but there is typically a rapidly growing and painful soft tissue mass together with a ragged area of radiolucency and variable radiopacity without definable pattern. Metastasis is mainly to the lungs (Fig. 116) producing cannon-ball radiopacities.

Microscopy

Appearances are variable and the tumour is either predominantly osteolytic (undifferentiated) or productive, and then may be predominantly osteochondroblastic or fibroblastic. It consists of abnormal neoplastic osteoblasts, which are typically angular, hyperchromatic and larger than normal; often in large numbers in some areas (Fig. 114). Tumour osteoid (Fig. 113) and bone are often formed and predominate in the osteoblastic type. Amounts may be small in the chondro- or fibroblastic variants. Sometimes the tumour is highly vascular or 'telangiectatic'. Surrounding normal bone is destroyed (Fig. 115).

Histological characteristics do not seem to correlate well with prognosis.

Treatment and prognosis

Osteosarcomas are highly malignant. Wide excision and chemotherapy may provide a 5-year survival rate of approximately 40% but deaths continue even after a decade.

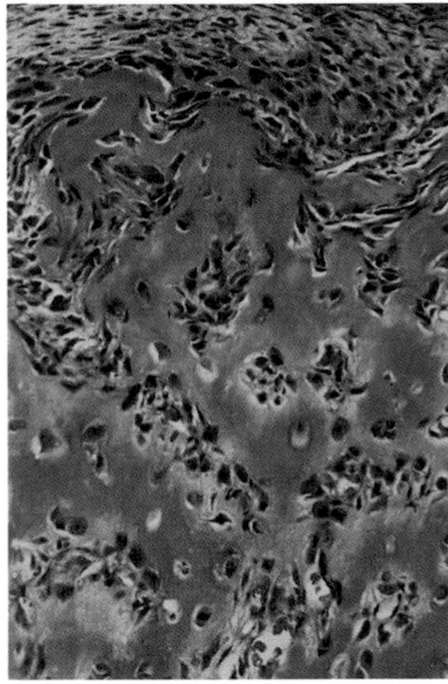

Fig. 113 Osteosarcoma with tumour osteoid.

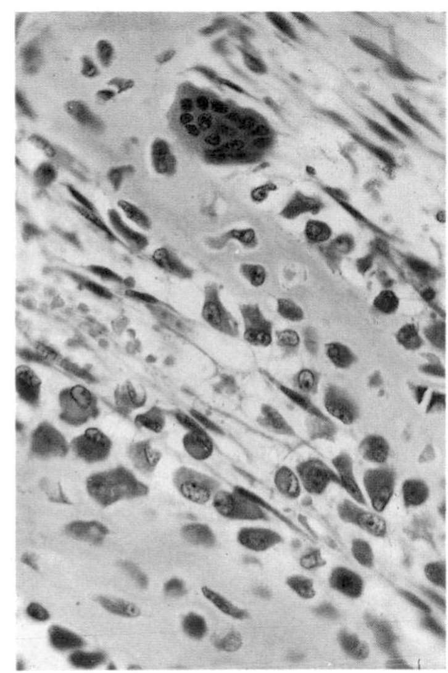

Fig. 114 Osteosarcoma: malignant osteoblasts.

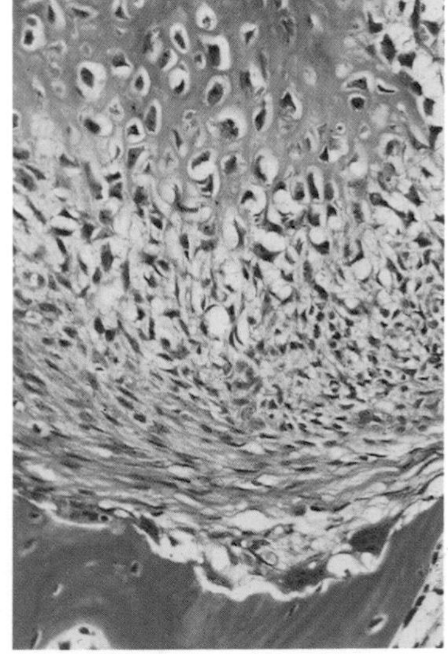

Fig. 115 Osteosarcoma: invasion of normal bone.

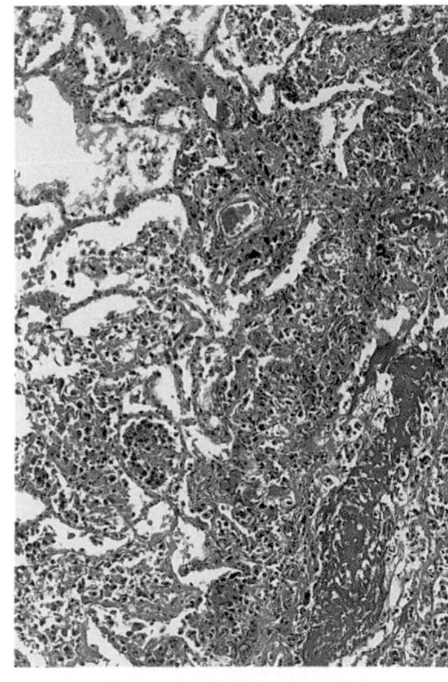

Fig. 116 Osteosarcoma: secondary in lung.

Central giant cell granuloma of the jaws

Aetiology

Unknown; *not* a neoplasm and *not* an osteoclastoma. It was mistakenly termed 'reparative giant cell granuloma' in the past (but it is more destructive than reparative). There is no evidence of traumatic aetiology and there are no changes in blood chemistry. Adolescents or young adults are mainly affected, especially females, the usual site being the mandible. The tumour produces an area of radiolucency often with faint trabeculation and indefinite borders or a soap bubble appearance.

Microscopy

Loose, usually highly cellular and vascular connective tissue stroma containing multinucleate giant cells of variable size (Figs 117 & 118). The lesions are not histologically distinguishable from bone lesions of hyperparathyroidism.

Behaviour

Occasionally there is rapid growth and corresponding extension of bone destruction, but the tumour is benign and responds to conservative resection. Residual areas may resolve spontaneously.

Multiple myeloma and solitary plasmacytoma

Myeloma is a malignant tumour of plasma cells causing multiple painful punched-out foci of bone destruction or pathological fractures. Solitary plasmacytomas are rare and may be in soft tissue. Most ultimately become multiple.

Occasionally, the condition is detected early, by chance finding of monoclonal hypergammaglobulinaemia during routine haematological investigation.

Microscopy

The neoplastic plasma cells (Fig. 119) produce monoclonal immunoglobulin—usually IgG. Amyloid formation (Fig. 120) both within the tumour and in other sites, such as the tongue, may result.

Prognosis

The median survival for multiple myeloma, even with chemotherapy, is 2–3 years. The 5-year survival rate is less than 20%. Solitary myelomas usually become multiple within 2–20 years.

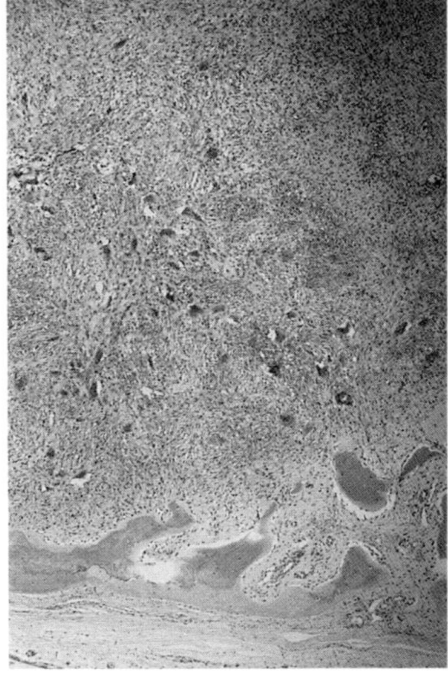

Fig. 117 Central giant cell granuloma.

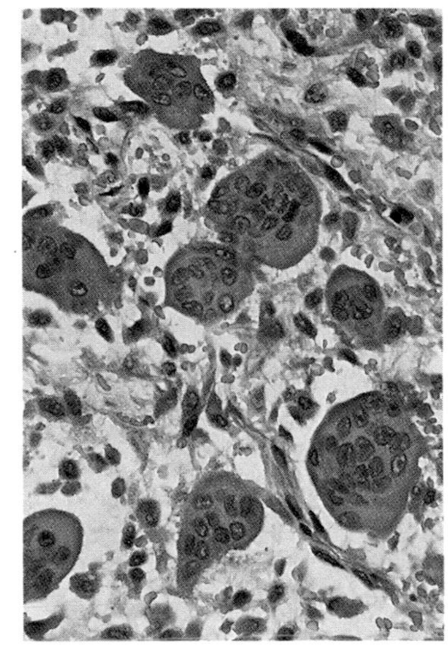

Fig. 118 Giant cell granuloma: typical 'osteoclasts'.

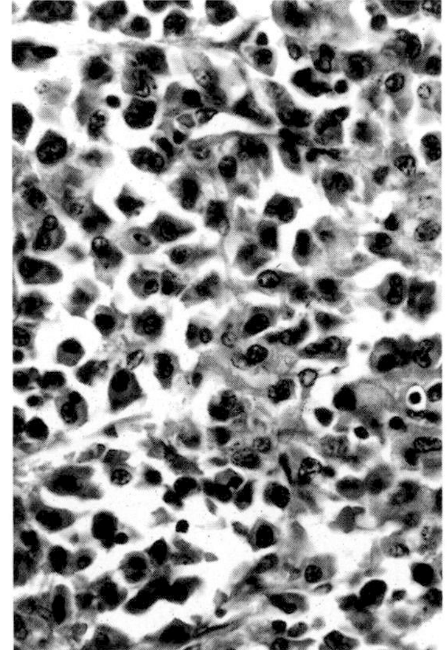

Fig. 119 Myeloma: tumour plasma cells.

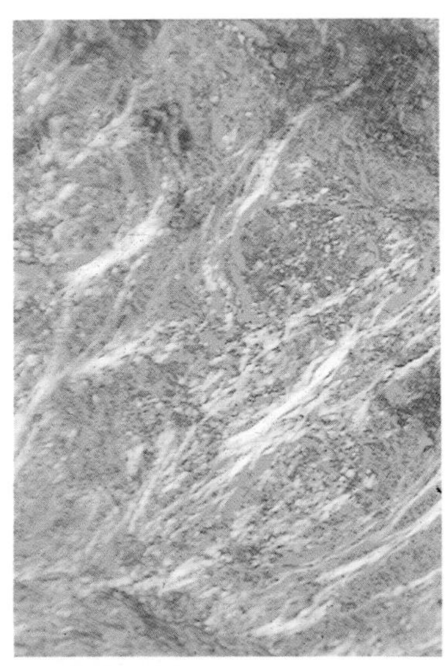

Fig. 120 Myeloma amyloid (green fluorescence with polarized light of Congo Red).

Langerhans cell histiocytosis (histiocytosis X; eosinophilic granuloma)

A rare tumour or tumour-like disease of the Langerhans cells (dendritic, antigen-presenting cells) causing solitary or multiple areas of destruction of bone and sometimes of periodontal tissues, exposing the roots of teeth. Eosinophilic granuloma may be solitary or multiple.

Microscopy

The mass consists of pleomorphic 'histiocytes' and eosinophils in dense clusters or thinly scattered (Fig. 121). 'Histiocytes' are typically large and pale and variable in size and shape (Fig. 122) with lobulated nuclei.

Hand–Schüller–Christian disease
Strictly, this is a triad of osteolytic lesions of the skull, exophthalmos and diabetes insipidus but the name is often applied to any type of multifocal eosinophilic granuloma. It is a rare variant.

Letterer–Siwe disease
This affects infants or young children. Typically, it also involves soft tissues (rashes, lymphadenopathy, splenomegaly, fever and anaemia). The prognosis is poor.

Prognosis

Isolated eosinophilic granuloma typically responds to curettage or may sometimes resolve spontaneously. In children with widespread disease, the disease is sometimes fatal despite chemotherapy.

Secondary tumours

Carcinomatous metastases are overall the most common tumours of bone but considerably less common in the jaws. Secondaries can come particularly from carcinomas of the breast, lung, prostate, thyroid or kidney and are recognizable by their resemblance to the primary tumour (Figs 123 & 124). A deposit in the jaw is very rarely the first sign of a distant asymptomatic primary.

Jaw metastases are typically a sign of disseminated disease and the prognosis is very poor.

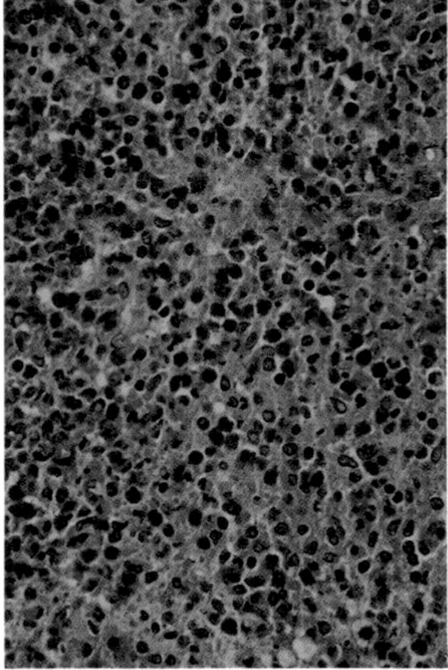

Fig. 121 Eosinophilic granuloma.

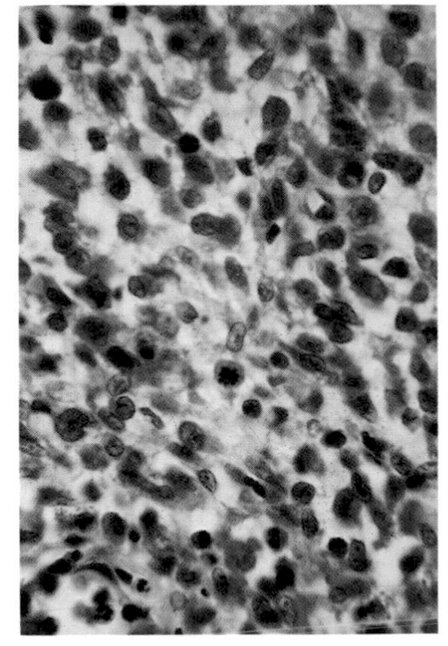

Fig. 122 Eosinophilic granuloma. (High power.)

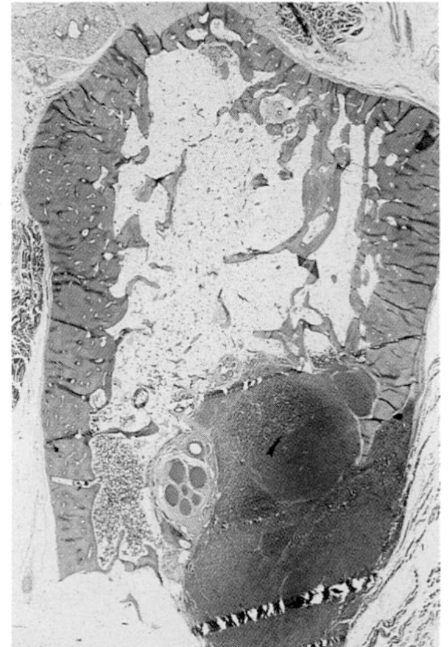

Fig. 123 Secondary carcinoma in mandible.

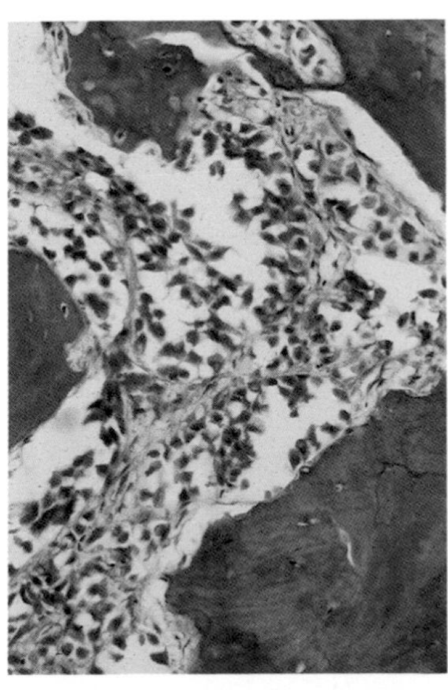

Fig. 124 Secondary deposit of bronchial carcinoma in jaw.

Fibrous dysplasia (monostotic)

Typically seen in young adults of either sex as rounded, painless, smooth bony swelling of the maxilla. The swelling may disturb function or occlusion.

Radiography shows a rounded area of relative radiolucency often with fine orange peel or ground glass appearance, but lesions vary from predominantly fibrous with pseudocystic appearance to patchily sclerotic, and densely ossified. **The borders merge imperceptibly with surrounding normal bone**.

Microscopy

Rounded mass of loose, cellular fibrous tissue, typically containing evenly distributed slender trabeculae of woven bone (Figs 125 & 126) with osteoblasts within them (Fig. 127), blending imperceptibly with normal bone trabeculae at margins. The amount of bone is highly variable. Sometimes small foci of scattered giant cells (Fig. 128) or myxoid tissue can be seen. There are no significant changes in blood chemistry.

Prognosis

Typically, there is a spontaneous arrest of progress with skeletal maturity. Resection is only required for disfigurement or disturbed function.

Polyostotic fibrous dysplasia

Onset is often in childhood, predominantly in females. There are multiple lesions with macular skin pigmentation, endocrine disturbances and precocious puberty in females in Albright syndrome.

Microscopy

Similar to monostotic type.

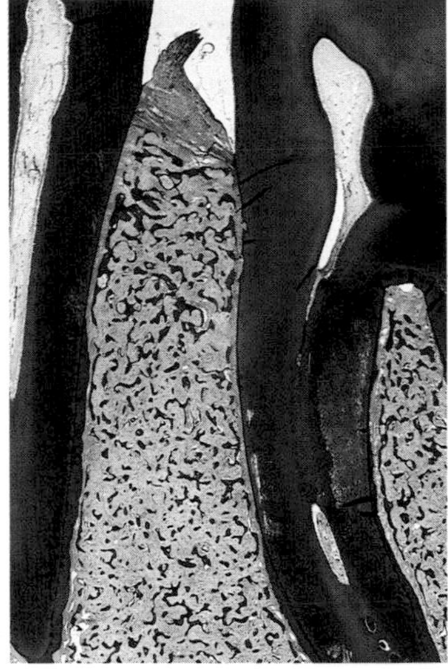

Fig. 125 Fibrous dysplasia involving periodontal tissues.

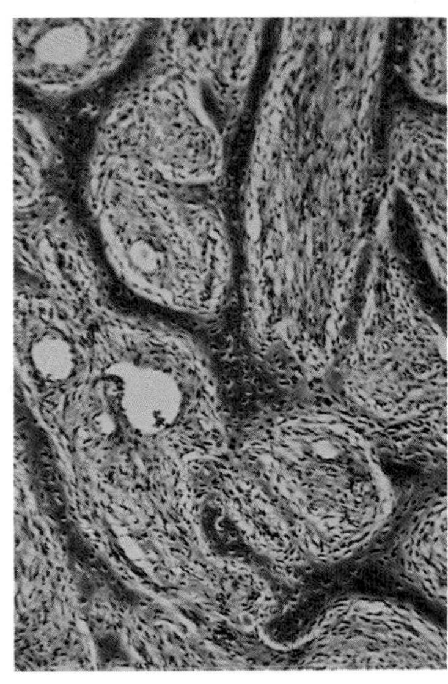

Fig. 126 Fibrous dysplasia: trabeculae of woven bone.

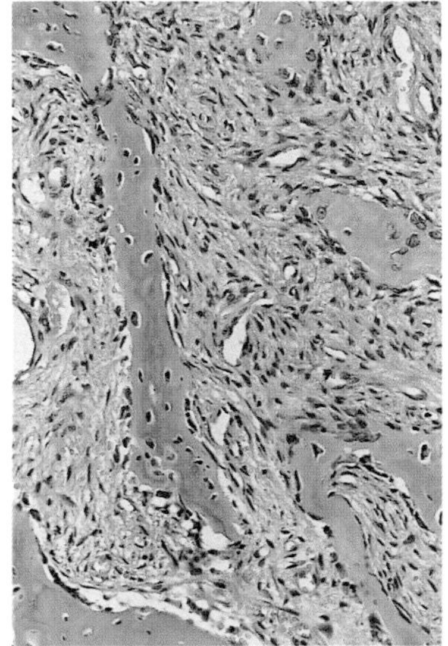

Fig. 127 Fibrous dysplasia: fine trabeculae of woven bone.

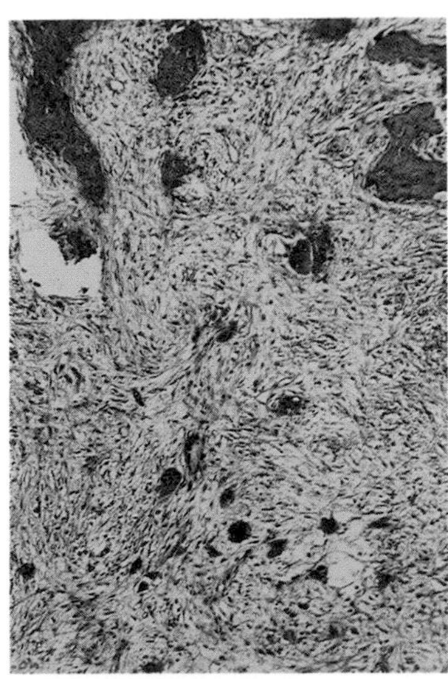

Fig. 128 Fibrous dysplasia: small focus of giant cells.

Cherubism (familial fibrous dysplasia)

Differs from fibrous dysplasia in:

- symmetrical involvement of jaws (mandible, ramus and adjacent body; maxillae also in severe cases) by giant cell lesions
- lesions appear multicystic on radiographs
- typically regresses with skeletal maturity
- autosomal dominant inheritance but poor penetration of the trait in females and many sporadic cases.

Radiolucencies precede swelling and may persist for some years after clinical resolution.

Microscopy

Replacement of bone by loose vascular connective tissue containing many giant cells usually resembling giant cell granuloma (Fig. 129). Histopathology of cherubism and fibrous dysplasia is not in itself diagnostic.

Confirmation depends on:

- clinical picture
- radiographic features
- behaviour of lesion.

Prognosis

Lesions typically regress completely with skeletal maturation. Treatment of active disease leads to recurrence.

Hyperparathyroidism

Aetiology

- Primary hyperparathyroidism—hypersecretion of parathormone by parathyroid tumour but bone lesions now exceedingly rare.
- Secondary hyperparathyroidism results from renal failure leading to reactive parathyroid hyperplasia.

Microscopy

Tumour-like foci of osteoclasts (Figs 130 & 131) produce cyst-like areas (sometimes multilocular) on radiographs (osteitis fibrosa cystica). Microscopically, the condition is indistinguishable from giant cell granuloma of the jaws. Diagnosis depends on serum chemistry changes, namely, raised calcium (up to ×2 normal), normal or low phosphate and raised alkaline phosphatase.

Prognosis

Removal of the parathyroid tumour leads to resolution of bone lesions.

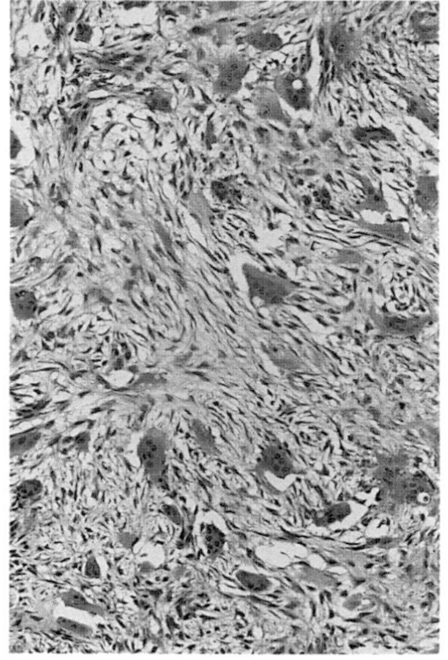

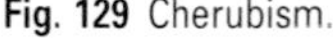

Fig. 129 Cherubism.

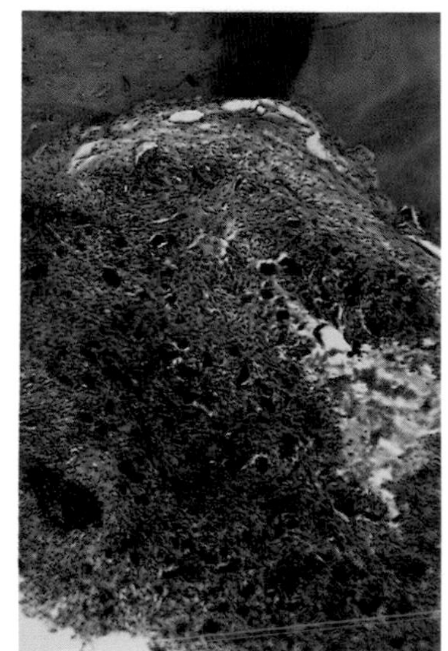

Fig. 130 Hyperparathyroidism.

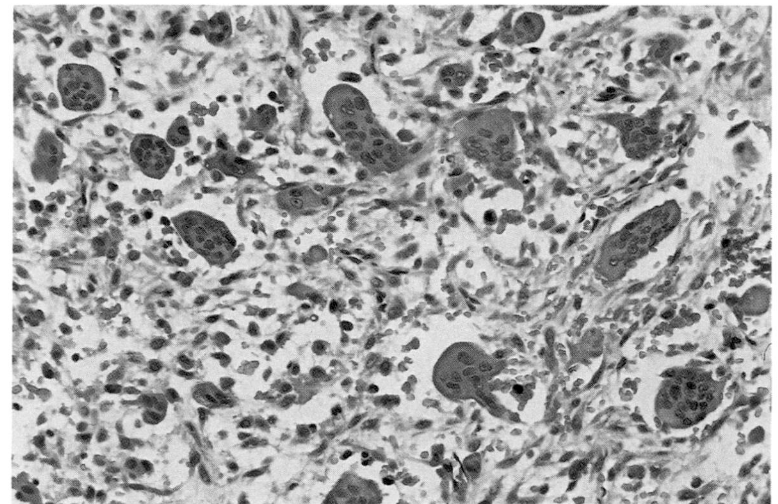

Fig. 131 Hyperparathyroidism: details of osteoclasts.

Paget's disease of bone (osteitis deformans)

Aetiology and prevalence

May be radiologically detectable in 5% of those over 55 in some areas of Britain, but symptomatic deforming disease is uncommon. The aetiology is unclear but there is evidence of weak genetic and possibly viral components.

The condition is usually polyostotic and most frequently affects the pelvis, calvarium and limbs. The maxilla is occasionally affected but the mandible only rarely. Lesions are predominantly osteolytic initially but there is increasing sclerosis, often with gross generalized thickening of bone. Alkaline phosphatase levels are greatly raised (up to ×20 normal).

Radiography. Variable radiolucency of the bone, with loss of trabeculation and lamina dura, followed by cotton-wool areas of radiopacity and gross, craggy hypercementosis. In the maxilla, gross thickening of the alveolar ridges causes the middle third of the face to bulge forward.

Microscopy

Anarchic disorganization of normal bone remodelling results in alternating resorption and deposition (Fig. 132): many osteoblasts and osteoclasts line the bone margins (Fig. 133). An irregular pattern of reversal lines produces a jigsaw-puzzle ('mosaic') pattern of basophilic lines in the bone, typically with predominant osteoclastic activity initially, but then with progressively increasing osteoblastic activity causing bones to become thicker and larger but weaker. Decreasing vascularity of bones in the late stages makes them susceptible to infection. Involvement of cementum produces craggy hypercementosis, which also shows a 'mosaic' pattern microscopically (Fig. 134).

Prognosis

The disease is typically active for 3–5 years but may then become virtually static but leaving persistent deformities.

Sarcomatous change in the axial skeleton is rare and virtually unknown in the jaws.

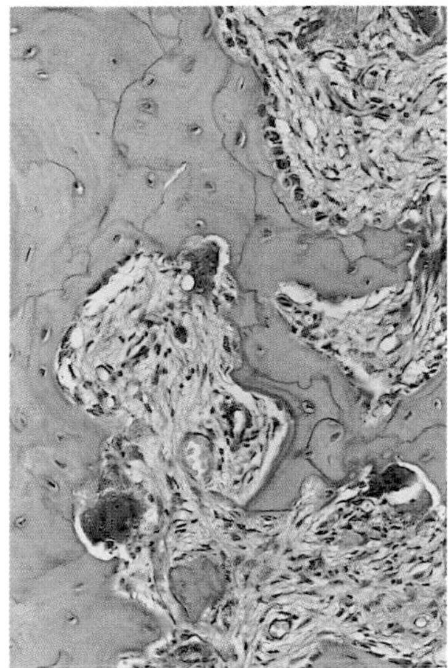

Fig. 132 Paget's disease. Reversal lines form a 'mosaic' pattern.

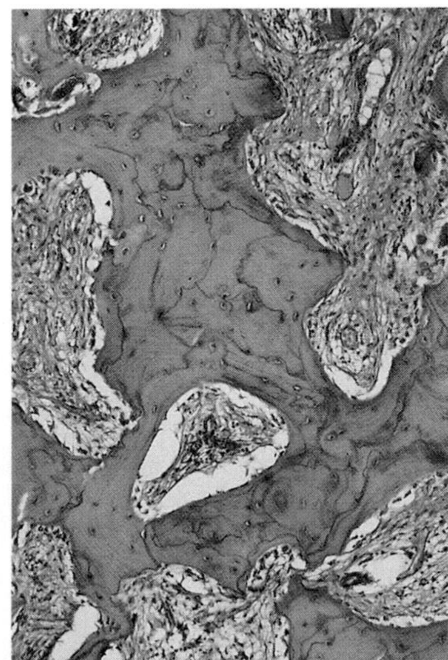

Fig. 133 Paget's disease of bone: 'mosaic' (reversal) lines.

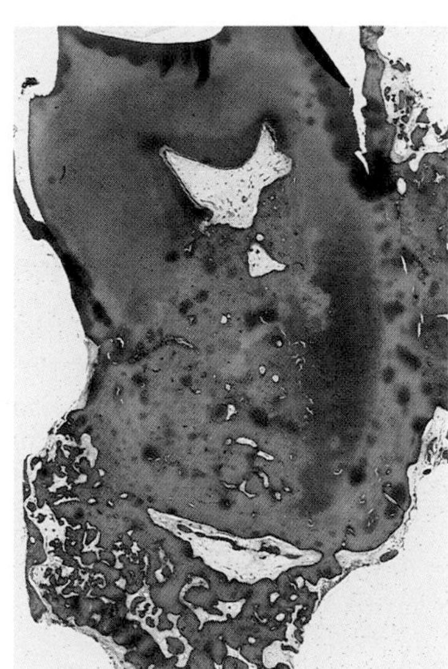

Fig. 134 Paget's disease: irregular hypercementosis of tooth.

Radiation injury (osteoradionecrosis)

Irradiation for cancer can cause death of bone cells leaving empty lacunae (Fig. 135) and obliterative endarteritis (Fig. 136), leaving severely ischaemic areas of bone. Attempts to separate this dead tissue by osteoclasts produce moth-eaten areas but this activity is limited by the poor blood supply. Infection, usually from teeth, readily spreads in the ischaemic bone and can give rise to extensive chronic osteomyelitis.

Osteomyelitis

Aetiology

Infection of the jaw can rarely result from severe dental infections or from fractures open to the skin, or it may be secondary to irradiation.

Microscopy

Infection spreads through the cancellous spaces leading to thrombosis of blood vessels in bony canaliculae and bone necrosis. Necrotic bone shows empty lacunae, is typically infiltrated by inflammatory cells (Figs 137 & 138) and may show masses of bacteria. Osteoclasts from healthy peripheral bone resorb the junction with infected bone which becomes separated as a sequestrum.

Prognosis

After confirming the bacterial cause with a specimen of pus, prompt, vigorous antibiotic treatment alone is usually effective. Sequestra are typically small and can be removed when loosened by resorption. Complications include progress to chronic osteomyelitis or spread of infection causing cellulitis or septicaemia but are rare.

Osteomyelitis after irradiation is chronic and difficult to eradicate. Hyperbaric oxygen therapy may be helpful. Occasionally it may be necessary to excise most of the jaw at its healthy margins.

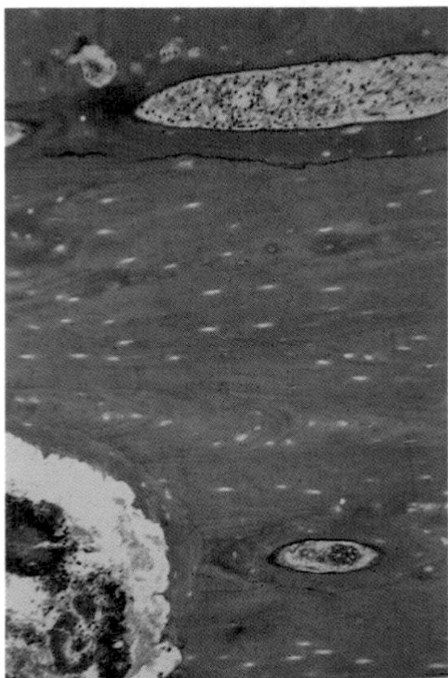

Fig. 135 Osteoradionecrosis.

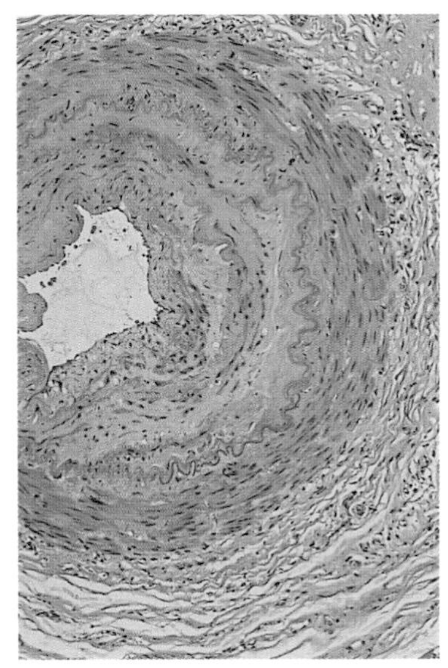

Fig. 136 Irradiation-induced obliterative endarteritis.

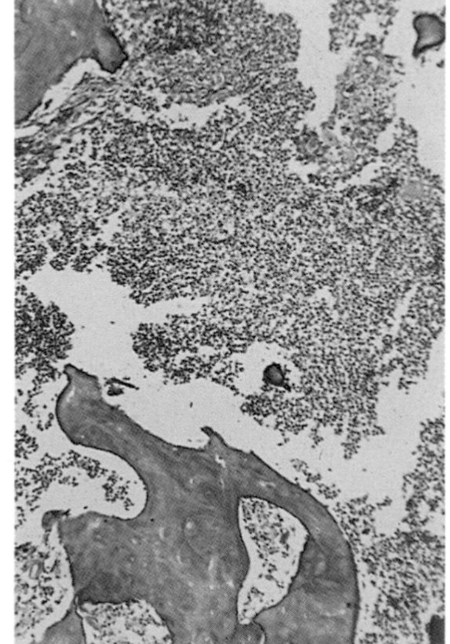

Fig. 137 Acute osteomyelitis: dead bone and inflammatory cells.

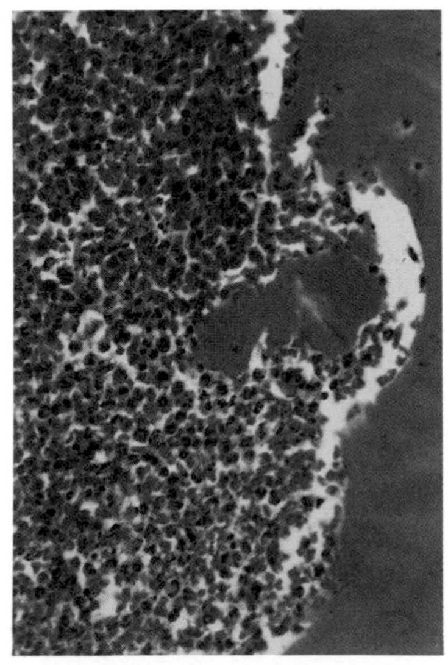

Fig. 138 Acute osteomyelitis: acute inflammatory cells in dead bone.

11 / Infective stomatitis

Herpetic stomatitis

Aetiology

A primary infection of a non-immune individual by HSV, usually type 1. Steadily declining incidence in developed countries but greater prevalence in immunodeficiency, e.g. AIDS.

Pathology

Viral infection of epithelial cells produces intra-epithelial vesicles (Fig. 139) with virus-damaged cells in the floor (Fig. 140) leading to epithelial destruction (Fig. 141), ulcers and inflammation.

Smears from early lesions show ballooning degeneration of epithelial cell nuclei (Fig. 142).

There is a systemic febrile illness, lymphadenopathy, and a rising titre of antibodies.

Oral lesions typically resolve within about a week but malaise may persist longer. Aciclovir mouth rinses may shorten the illness.

Herpes labialis

Virus may persist in the trigeminal ganglion. Periodic reactivation leads to vesicles and crusting ulcers on borders of lips in about 30% of patients after primary infection. Microscopic features are the same as for primary infection.

Herpes labialis typically resolves in about a week but very early application of aciclovir cream may abort an attack.

Herpes zoster of the trigeminal area

Aetiology

Reactivation of Varicella-zoster infection, usually in the elderly long after the initial infection (chickenpox). The condition is especially common and severe in immunodeficiencies; life-threatening in AIDS.

Trigeminal zoster affects the sensory area of skin and mucosa of the affected division, usually unilaterally and typically with aching pain.

Microscopy

Vesiculation and ulceration, the same as for herpes simplex.

Zoster is a disabling disease in the elderly and requires treatment with aciclovir.

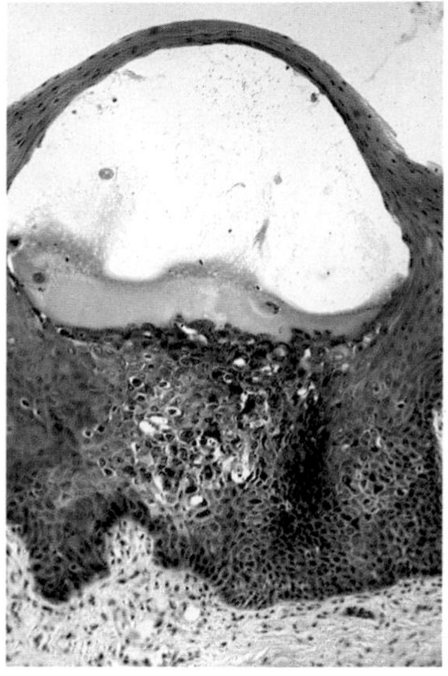

Fig. 139 Herpetic stomatitis: intact vesicle.

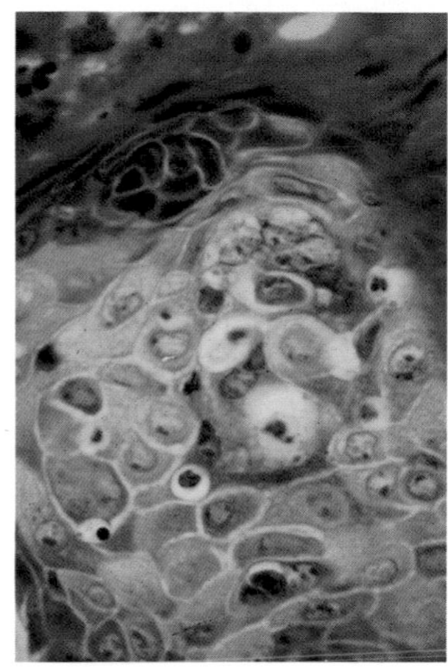

Fig. 140 Herpetic stomatitis: virus-damaged cells in floor of vesicle.

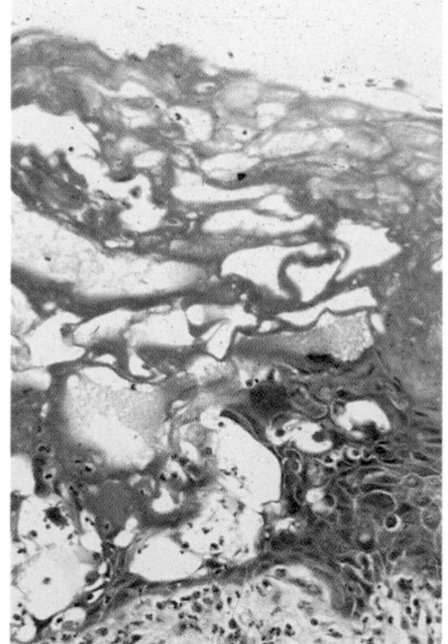

Fig. 141 Herpetic stomatitis: necrosis of epithelium.

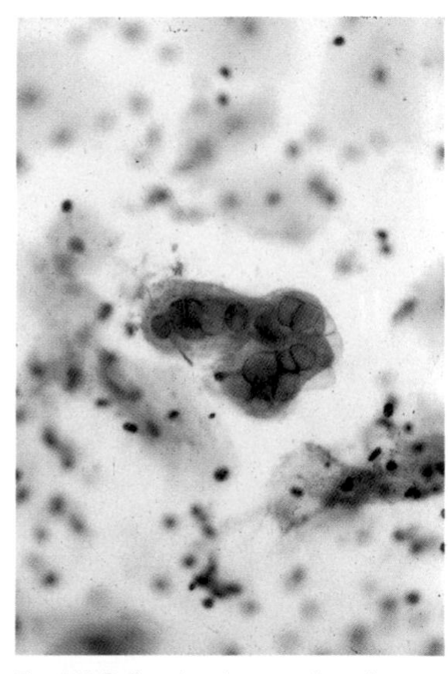

Fig. 142 Ballooning degeneration of epithelial cells in smear.

12 / Non-infective stomatitis

Non-specific ulceration can result from trauma or unidentified causes as in recurrent aphthae.

Recurrent aphthae

Aetiology

Unknown in most cases. Many reported immunological abnormalities, but their aetiological significance is doubtful. This is not an autoimmune disease—it affects otherwise healthy persons, and is not associated with recognized autoimmune diseases. There are no useful immunological diagnostic tests and there is no reliable response to immunosuppressive treatment.

In 5–10%, ulcers are precipitated by deficiency of, and respond to administration of, folate, vitamin B_{12} or occasionally iron.

From 10–20% of the population are affected in some degree. Typically ulceration starts mildly in childhood or adolescence, often peaks in early adult life and then gradually declines. Rare onset late in life is usually associated with a haematinic deficiency state.

Major aphthae, aphthae-like ulcers or ragged necrotizing mucosal ulcers are sometimes a feature of HIV infection.

Microscopy

Ulceration appears to be preceded by leucocytic infiltration of the epithelium and underlying corium and intercellular oedema leading to disintegration of the epithelium (Fig. 143). Ulcers have no specific features but consist of a break in the epithelium with an intense inflammatory infiltrate extending deeply (Fig. 144). Diagnosis therefore depends largely on the history of regular recurrences and clinical features.

Behaviour and prognosis

There is no consistently effective treatment for common aphthae but treatment with topical corticosteroids, for example, may ameliorate the condition.

Major aphthae, particularly in patients with AIDS, may require treatment with and respond to thalidomide.

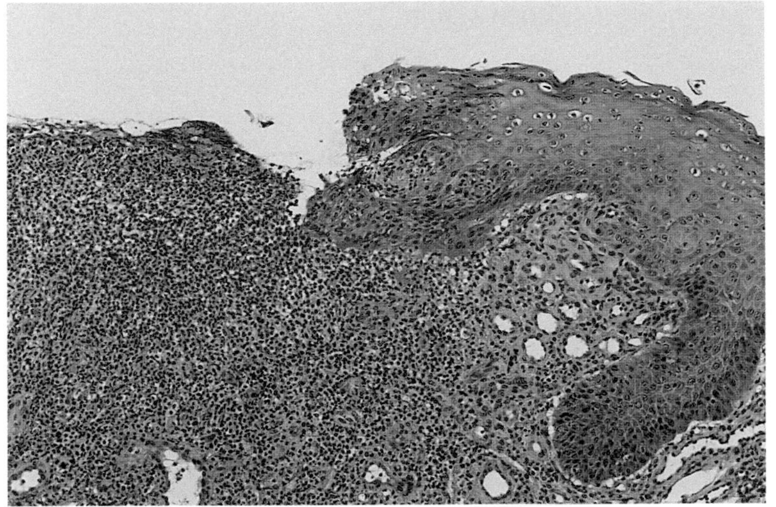

Fig. 143 Aphtha: margin of an active ulcer.

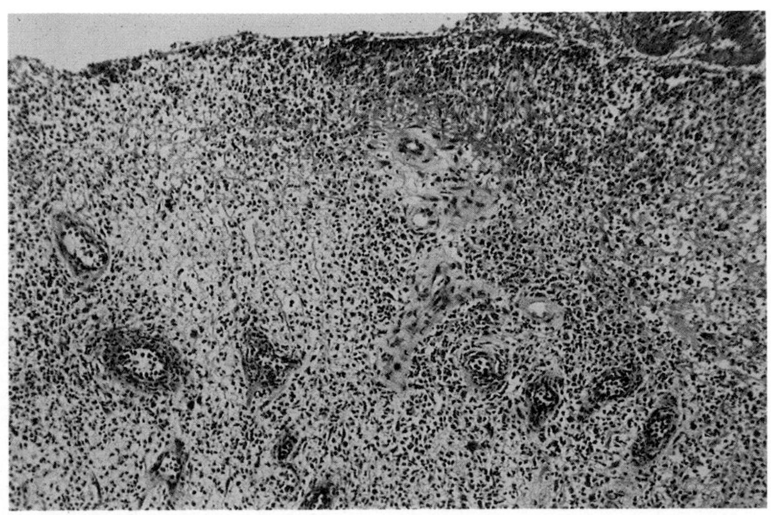

Fig. 144 Aphtha: centre of ulcer.

Lichen planus

Aetiology

Unknown, but some cases are drug induced. Immunological damage to the epithelium is suggested by the predominantly T lymphocyte infiltrate but no reason for the lymphocytotoxic reaction has been convincingly demonstrated. The disease affects otherwise healthy persons and is not associated with typical autoimmune diseases. It is most common after the age of 45; about 65% of cases are in females. The most frequent clinical manifestation is a lacy pattern of *white striae* on the buccal mucosa, typically symmetrically. Other sites include the margins and dorsum of the tongue or, infrequently, the gingivae (usually atrophic areas, rarely striae). *Atrophic lesions* are red and smooth. *Erosions* typically have depressed margins and may be covered by a raised layer of yellowish fibrin. White plaques mainly result from longstanding disease. Cutaneous lichen planus is frequently not associated.

Microscopy

The inflammatory infiltrate consists mainly of CD4 and CD8 T lymphocytes. However, CD8 T-cells are more numerous in relation to the epithelium and their numbers rise with disease activity.

Striae (white lesions). Hyper- or parakeratosis is associated with pointed, sometimes saw-tooth rete ridges, liquefaction degeneration of the basal cell layer (see Fig. 148, p. 80) and a band-like mononuclear (predominantly T lymphocyte) infiltrate with a well-defined lower border in the corium (Figs 145 & 146). These 'classical' changes rarely seen together.

Atrophic (red) lesions. The epithelium is thin and flattened without keratosis. The inflammatory infiltrate is more dense but still band-like (Fig. 147).

Erosions. The epithelium is destroyed by progression of atrophy (**not** by rupture of bullae). Secondary infection increases the inflammatory response and produces a non-specific picture apart from any changes of lichen planus at the margins. ➡

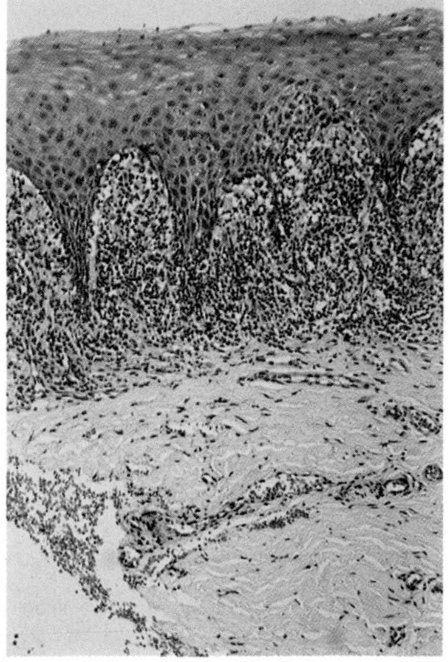

Fig. 145 Lichen planus.

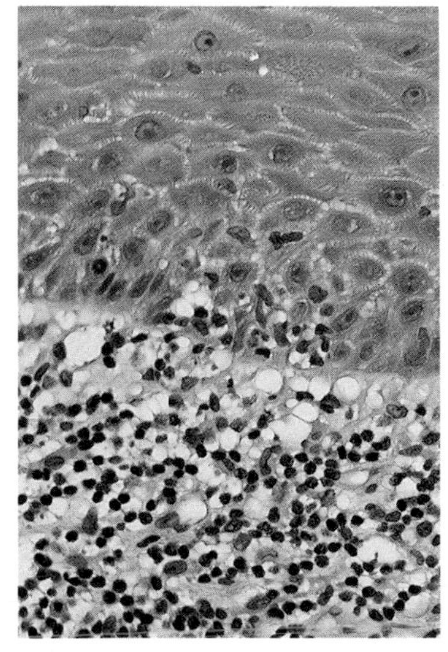

Fig. 146 Lichen planus: detail of liquefaction degeneration of basal cells.

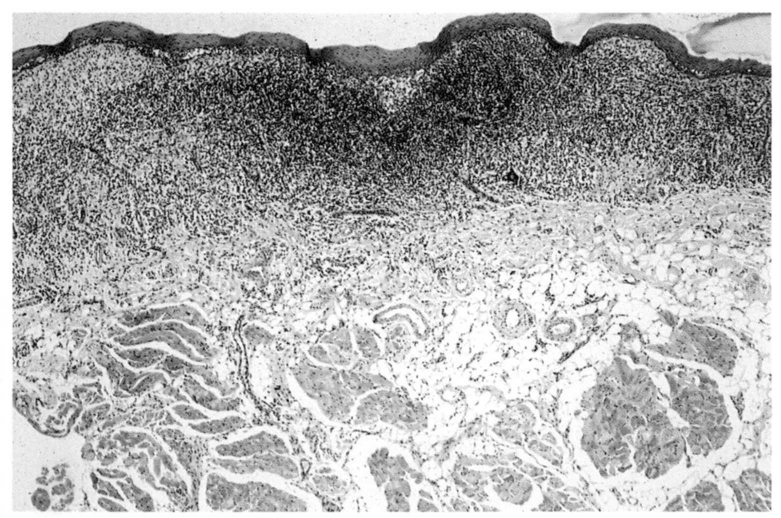

Fig. 147 Lichen planus: atrophic type.

Treatment and prognosis

Lichen planus, though usually self-limiting, can persist for many years if untreated. Frequently, there is a good response to topical corticosteroids: systemic corticosteroids are usually effective if topical treatment fails. Approximately 1% risk of malignant change over a 10-year period for specific sites.

Lichenoid reactions

The term *lichenoid* reactions sometimes causes considerable confusion, and the relationship between lichen planus, drug-induced lichen planus and other lichen planus-like reactions is unclear.

Lichenoid reactions to drugs, amalgams or other restorative materials can sometimes present 'classical' features of lichen planus histologically and there is considerable overlap between the histological appearances of classical lichen planus and lichenoid reactions.

Some drug-induced and other lichenoid reactions show greater numbers of plasma cells superficially in the corium. Perivascular inflammatory infiltrates and formation of deep lymphoid follicles also suggest a topical or systemic drug reaction.

Histologically, lichenoid reactions to amalgam can appear the same as those of idiopathic lichen planus or occasionally similar to those of drug reactions. Alternatively, there may be prominent lymphoid follicles, neutrophils in the epithelium and, sometimes, epithelial atypia (Figs 149 & 150).

In view of the difficulty of distinguishing idiopathic from iatrogenic lichen planus histologically, the diagnosis can be made only with the establishment of a drug history or of contact of the lesion with a restoration. Confirmation depends on resolution following withdrawal of the drug or replacement of the restoration.

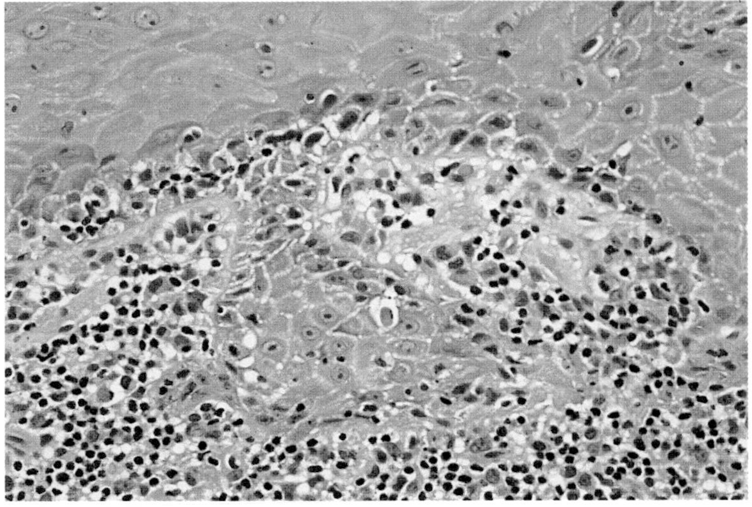

Fig. 148 Lichen planus, basal cell degeneration (apoptoses).

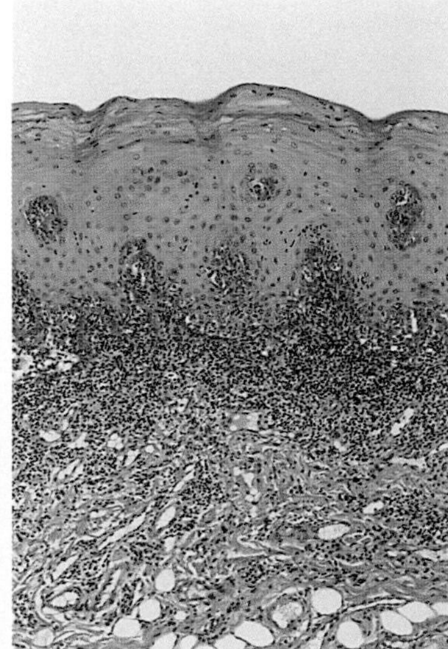

Fig. 149 Lichenoid reaction.

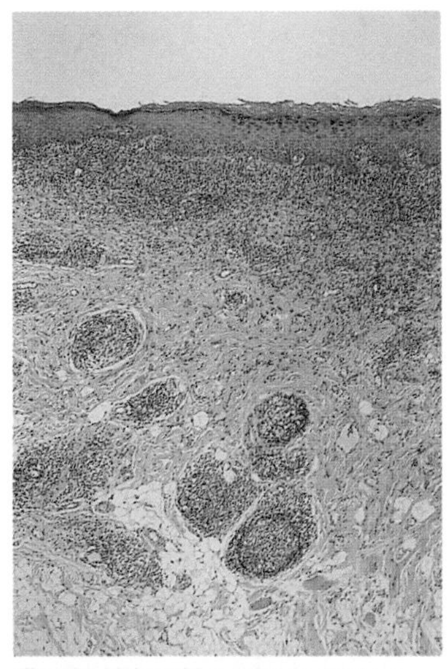

Fig. 150 Lichenoid reaction to amalgam with deep lymphoid follicles.

Bullous erythema multiforme (Stevens–Johnson syndrome)

Aetiology

Unknown, but occasionally follows drug treatment (especially long-acting sulphonamides) or herpetic or mycoplasmal infection (primary atypical pneumonia). However, no triggering factor is identifiable in most cases. No immunological mechanism has been identified.

The disease typically affects young adults and tends to recur 2 or 3 times a year and then spontaneously resolves after a time.

Pathology

This is a mucocutaneous vesiculobullous disease but orolabial lesions alone are common. Rarely, recently ruptured bullae are seen on the lips but not in the mouth. Clinically, swollen, bleeding and crusted lips are a typical feature. Oral ulceration is often widespread but ill-defined and nondescript in character. Target lesions or bullae affect the skin, and conjunctivitis or iritis may be associated.

Microscopy

Variable picture with degeneration of spinous cells and widespread intercellular oedema, sometimes leading to intra-epithelial vesiculation or extensive vacuolar change leading to subepithelial vesiculation (Figs 151 & 152).

Rupture of vesicles leaves erosions. There is a mononuclear inflammatory infiltrate subepithelially and around superficial blood vessels (Fig. 153).

Prognosis

Orofacial erythema multiforme tends to recur 2–3 times a year but frequently resolves after a few years. If severe it may respond to systemic corticosteroids or sometimes to aciclovir. Rarely, it progresses to potentially fatal multisystem disease with malaise and fever and toxic epidermal necrolysis or fatal renal disease.

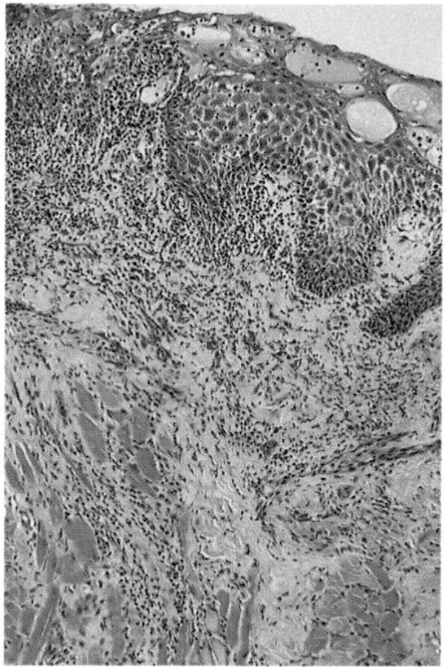

Fig. 151 Bullous erythema multiforme, early stage.

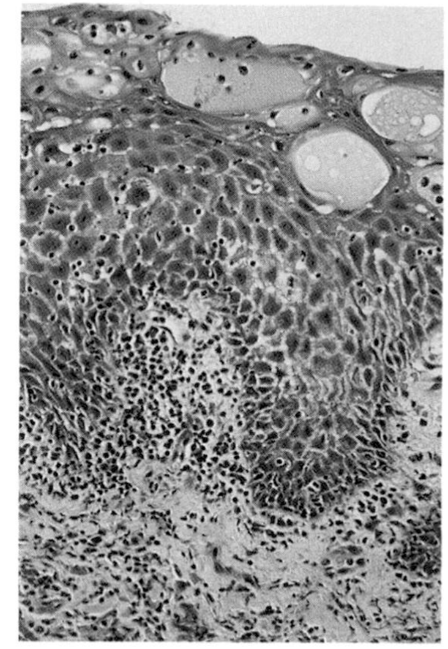

Fig. 152 Erythema multiforme: higher power.

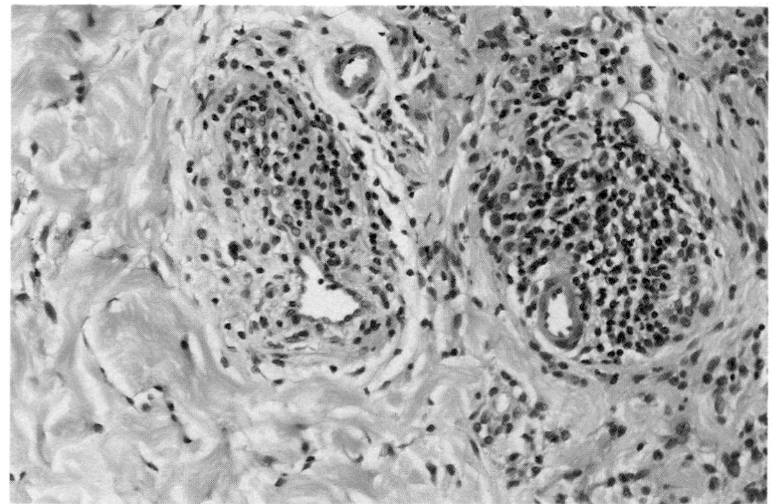

Fig. 153 Erythema multiforme: perivascular inflammatory infiltrate.

Pemphigus vulgaris

Aetiology and pathology

A 'typical' autoimmune disease with circulating autoantibodies against the epithelial intercellular adhesion molecule, desmoglein 3, which can be demonstrated in situ by immunofluorescence. Destruction of intercellular adherence leads to disintegration of epithelia and intra-epithelial vesiculation, often first in the mouth.

Clinically, women are more frequently affected, usually between the ages of 40 and 50, sometimes with oral lesions as the first sign. Vesicles are fragile, rarely seen intact in the mouth, but they typically leave small, painful irregular erosions. Occasionally, vesicles are produced by stroking the mucosa (Nikolsky's sign). Bullae are obvious on skin and can spread over the whole body. Rupture leaves crusted lesions.

Microscopy

Separation of epithelial cells from one another (acantholysis) initially forming suprabasal clefts then intra-epithelial vesicles. Basal cells adhere to one another and to underlying connective tissue to form the floor of vesicles but they eventually separate after rupture of vesicles (Fig. 154) to leave ulcers with inflammatory infiltrate in the floor. Prickle cells after acantholysis become rounded, float off in vesicle fluid (Fig. 155) and are seen in smears (Tzanck cells).

There is positive immunofluorescence of immunoglobulin (usually IgG) along intercellular junctions and coating detached acantholytic cells.

Absolute confirmation of the diagnosis is possible by immunofluorescence for immunoglobulin (Fig. 156), but histology is frequently adequate.

Prognosis

Cutaneous fluid and electrolyte loss or infection are usually fatal if untreated. Immunosuppressive treatment is life-saving but heavy doses of corticosteroids and azathioprine are required. Relapse frequently follows withdrawal of treatment but deaths are mainly a complication of immunosuppression and frequently result from infection. The overall mortality long term is about 6%.

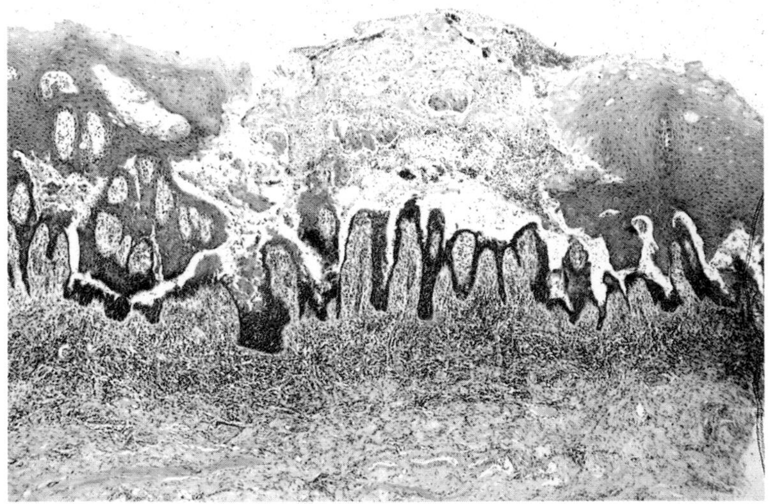

Fig. 154 Pemphigus vulgaris: recently ruptured vesicle.

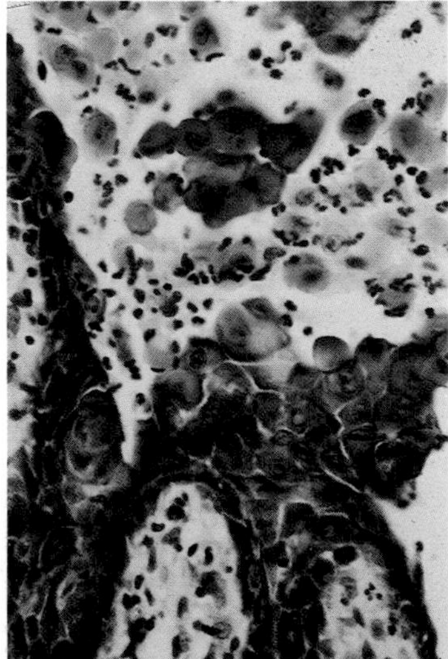

Fig. 155 Pemphigus vulgaris: acantholytic cells separating from each other—early stage.

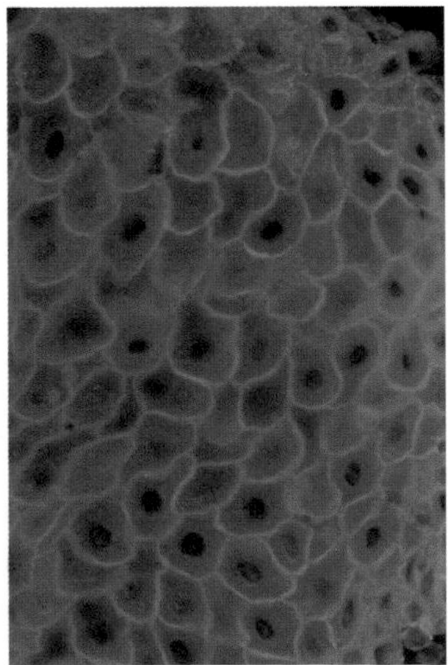

Fig. 156 Pemphigus vulgaris: immunofluorescence showing binding of antibody to intercellular adhesion molecules.

Mucous membrane pemphigoid

Aetiology and pathology

There is some evidence for immunopathogenesis with formation of antibodies against the basement membrane zone (BMZ). Women are mainly affected between the ages of 50–70 years.

Bullae and vesicles result from loss of attachment of epithelium to the underlying connective tissue. Bullae result from minor trauma; Nikolsky's sign may be positive; ruptured vesicles leave indolent erosions; lesions on gingivae may be called 'desquamative gingivitis'. Scarring (and damage to sight) is common in the ocular variant but rare in the mouth.

Microscopy

- Subepidermal bulla separating full thickness of epithelium from lamina propria.
- No acantholysis.
- Mixed, chronic inflammatory infiltrate in lamina propria (Figs 157 & 158).

Electron microscopy shows the level of separation of the epithelium to be along the lamina lucida (between the plasma membrane of the basal cells and the electron-dense basal lamina).

Autoantibodies to basement membrane zone material (anti-BMZ ab) are not routinely detectable in serum: immunofluorescence to immunoglobulins along the BMZ is seen in about 40% but the complement component (C_3) is seen in about 80% (see Fig. 159, p. 88). There is a poor correlation between anti-BMZ ab titres and the severity of the disease as assessed by routine methods. There is no recognized association with other more typical autoimmune diseases.

Prognosis

The disease is persistent but benign and oral lesions frequently respond to topical corticosteroids. Systemic steroids may sometimes be required particularly for ocular involvement.

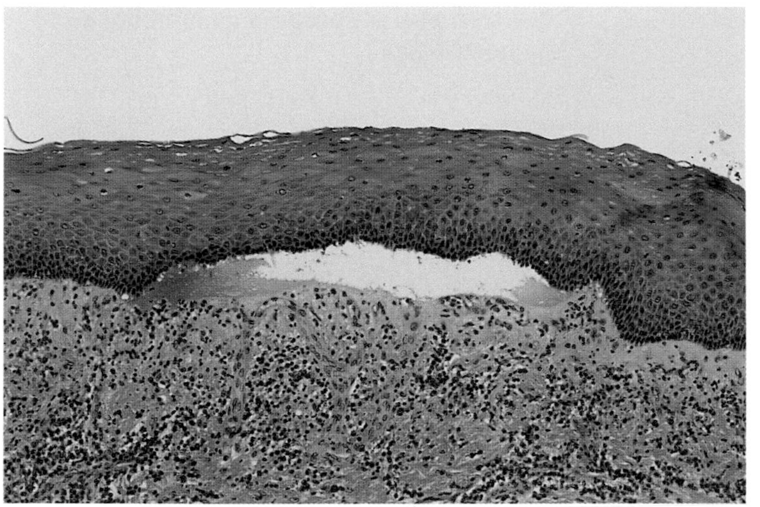

Fig. 157 Mucous membrane pemphigoid. Separation of full thickness of the epithelium from the corium.

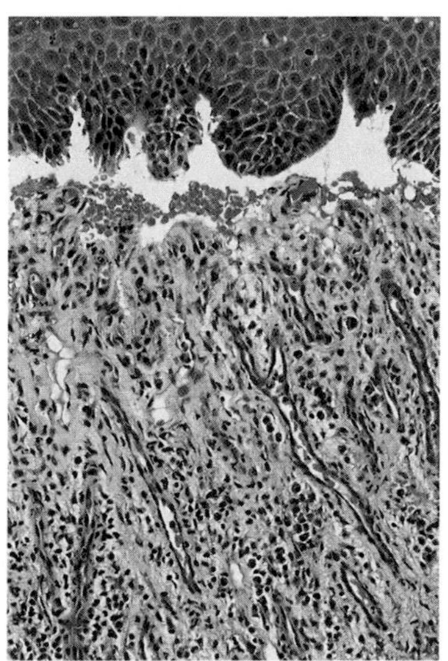

Fig. 158 Mucous membrane pemphigoid. (High power.)

Localized oral purpura ('angina bullosa haemorrhagica')

Purpura localized to the oral cavity (i.e. in the absence of a haemostatic defect) causes blood blisters, probably because of some local defect of blood vessels. Rupture of the roof of the blister leaves a painful ulcer. In the throat this can cause a choking sensation ('angina') (Fig. 160).

Localized oral purpura must be distinguished from the blisters of pemphigoid which sometimes fill with blood.

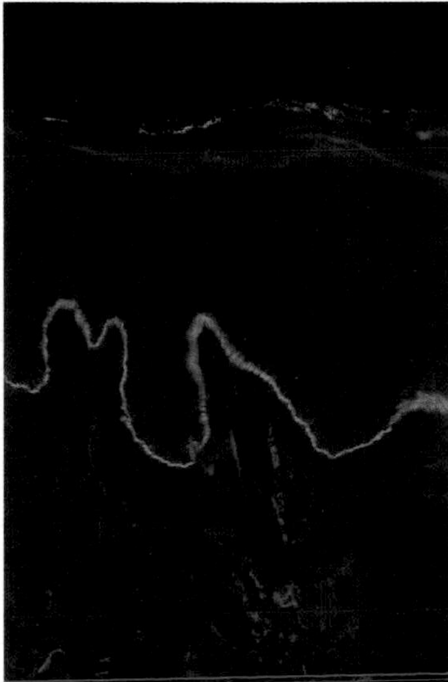

Fig. 159 Mucous membrane pemphigoid: immunofluorescence of complement (C_3) along basement membrane zone.

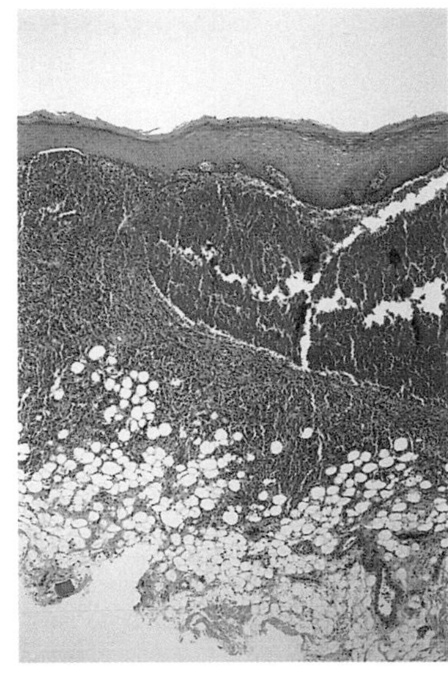

Fig. 160 Localized oral purpura. Blood blister due to subepithelial leakage of blood.

Lupus erythematosus

Aetiology and pathology

Either systemic or discoid lupus erythematosus (SLE or DLE) can cause oral lesions.

SLE is a connective tissue disease (autoimmune), thought to be immune-complex mediated, with multiple non-organ-specific autoantibodies, particularly antinuclear factors and often rheumatoid factor. Common effects are rashes and arthritis but almost any system can be involved and Sjögren syndrome is present in about 30% of cases.

DLE is mucocutaneous with lesions appearing the same as those of SLE, but minimal systemic effects or autoantibody production.

Women aged 20–40 years are mainly affected. Oral lesions consist of streaky white or erythematous areas, or erosions frequently similar to those of lichen planus.

Microscopy

Highly variable picture with highly irregular patterns of acanthosis or epithelial atrophy, liquefaction degeneration of the basal cell layer and widely scattered inflammatory infiltrate in the corium (Figs 161 & 162). Thickening of the basement membrane zone is shown by PAS staining (Fig. 163). Immunoglobulin and complement are also detectable there by immunofluorescence.

Diagnosis of SLE should be confirmed by autoantibody studies, which differentiate it from DLE.

Treatment

Lesions often respond poorly to topical corticosteroids, but systemic corticosteroids are justifiable for extensive SLE.

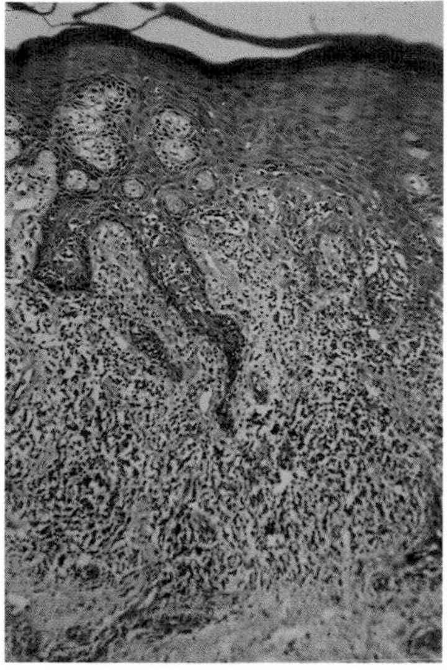

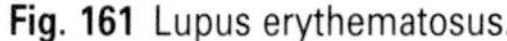

Fig. 161 Lupus erythematosus.

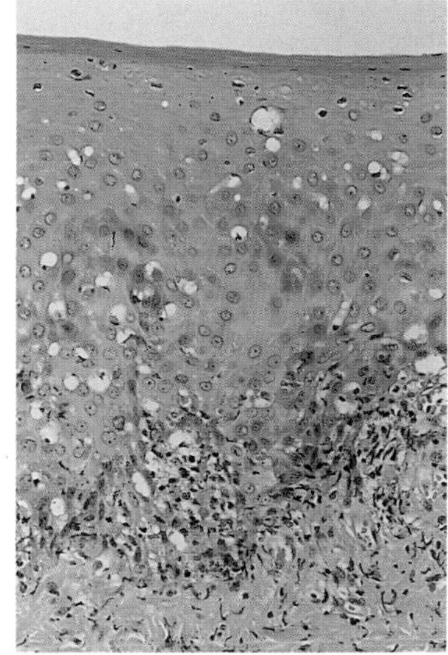

Fig. 162 Lupus erythematosus.

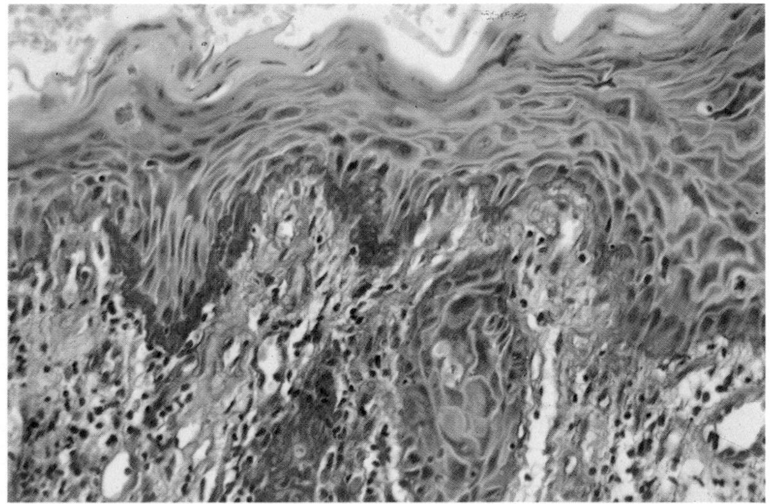

Fig. 163 Lupus erythematosus: basement membrane deposits of antigen/antibody. (PAS stain.)

13 / Keratoses (leukoplakias; white lesions)

Leukoplakias are chronic white (keratotic) mucosal plaques which are not due to any identifiable disease. The term is purely clinical and has no histological implications, but histology is necessary to exclude malignancy or other diseases. Most leukoplakias are not premalignant but red lesions (erythroplasias; p. 107) are frequently severely dysplastic or invasive carcinoma.

Terminology

Oral white plaques share many histological features, and idiopathic forms are often not distinguishable histologically from those with defined causes such as frictional keratosis, but may show dysplasia microscopically. Features of oral white lesions include the following in varying combinations:

Microscopy

- *Hyper(ortho)keratosis*: a superficial eosinophilic layer of dead epithelial squames under which there is a layer of epithelial cells containing basophilic granules of prekeratin (Fig. 164).
- *Parakeratosis*: the surface consists of effete epithelial cells containing shrunken, pyknotic, basophilic nuclei with no underlying granular cell layer (Figs 165 & 166).
- *Acanthosis*: hyperplasia of the prickle cell layer usually with loss of the normally regular profile of the rete ridges (Fig. 165).
- *Epithelial atrophy*: thinning usually with loss of the rete ridges of the epithelium (Fig. 167).
- *Dysplasia* (see pp. 105–106) may be associated with keratosis but there is no consistent relationship.

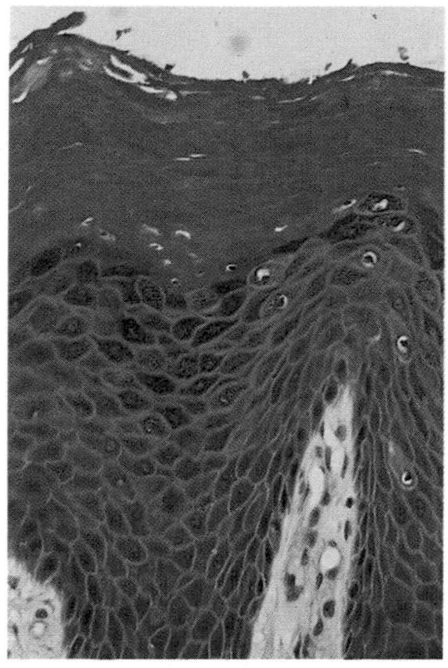

Fig. 164 Hyper(ortho)keratosis.

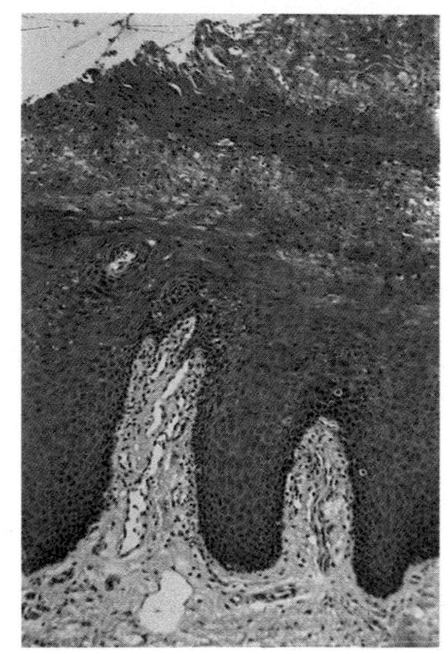

Fig. 165 Parakeratosis and acanthosis.

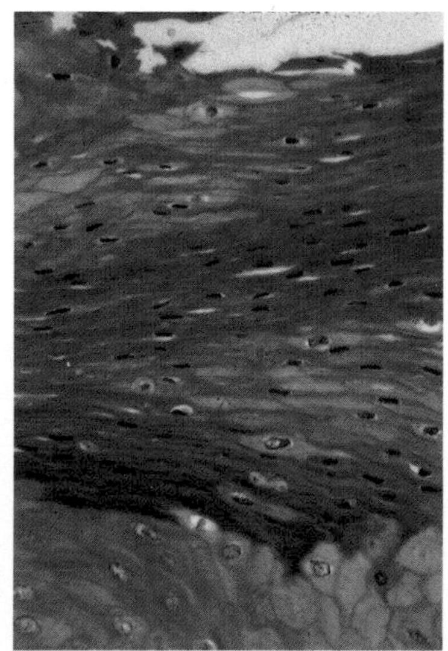

Fig. 166 Parakeratosis: detail.

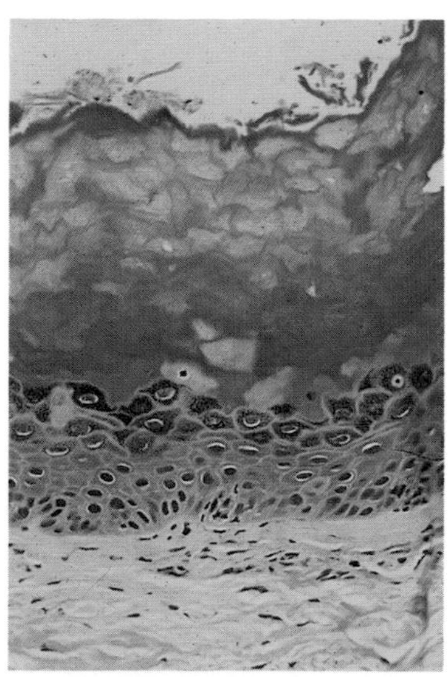

Fig. 167 Hyperorthokeratosis and epithelial atrophy.

White sponge naevus

Aetiology and pathology

Hereditary (autosomal dominant) disorder producing soft, white thickening of the oral mucosa. The condition is asymptomatic (may not be noticed until adulthood), but tags of protruding epithelium may be chewed off or detached, producing an irregular surface. The whole of the oral mucosa may be affected to variable degree.

Microscopy

Typically regular acanthosis with widespread intracellular oedema extending particularly in the plaque where prominent cell membranes give a 'basket-weave' appearance (Figs 168 & 169). The surface is typically irregular. Inflammatory infiltrate is absent from the corium (Fig. 170).

Prognosis

The condition is benign and once the diagnosis is confirmed by histology, only reassurance is required.

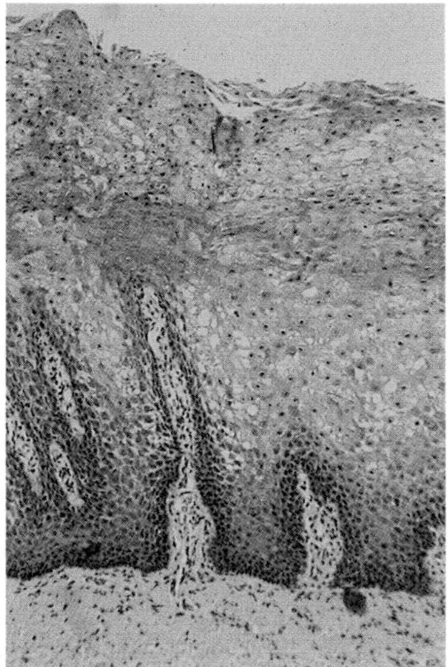

Fig. 168 White sponge naevus.

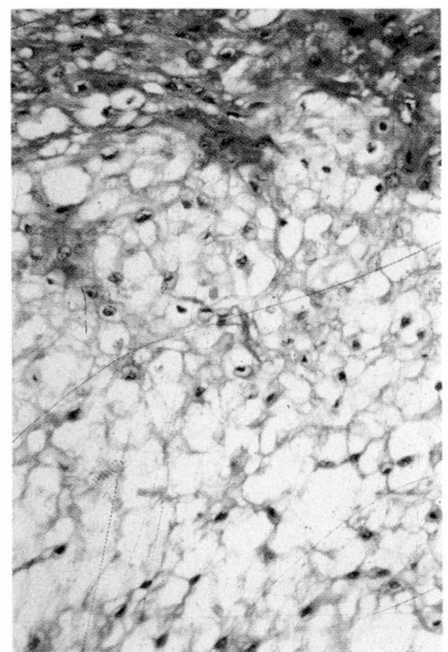

Fig. 169 White sponge naevus: oedematous epithelial cells.

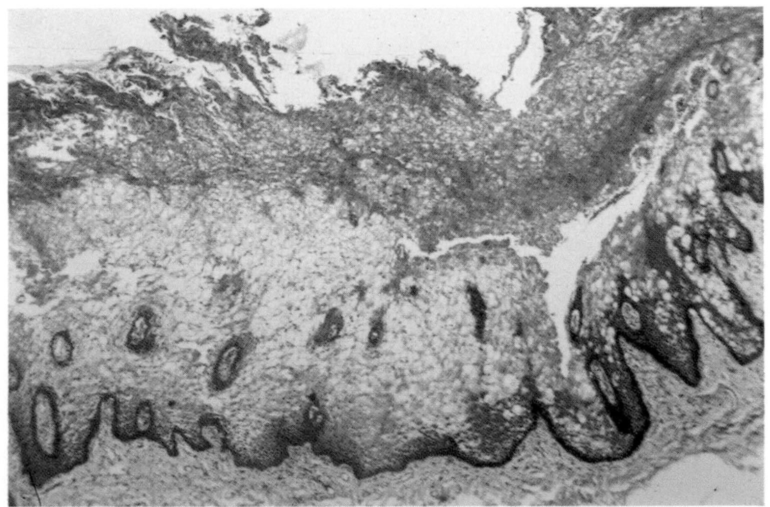

Fig. 170 White sponge naevus: partial detachment of plaque.

Leukoedema

Leukoedema is an anatomical variation consisting of a translucent, filmy thickening of the mucosa, most common in blacks.

Microscopy

Frequently, mild acanthosis with vacuolation of the superficial prickle cells (Fig. 171) gives a mild basket weave appearance, but less extensive than that seen in white sponge naevus (see Fig. 168, p. 94).

Behaviour and prognosis

Leukoedema is of no clinical significance.

Cheek-biting

Cheek-biting is a moderately common habit which may be a response to anxiety or used during periods of mental concentration. Clinically the buccal mucosa appears rough, with red areas and small tags of white thickened mucosa.

Microscopy

There is acanthosis and a thick, ragged parakeratinized layer on which there may be conspicuous bacterial colonization (Fig. 172). Occasionally the epithelium may contain koilocyte-like cells (Fig. 172) and bear some resemblance to hairy leukoplakia. However, the clinical features are significantly different.

Behaviour and prognosis

Clinically, cheek-biting is of little clinical significance, though it may be confused with other white patches. The patient may require reassurance and be advised to be aware of the needlessness of the habit.

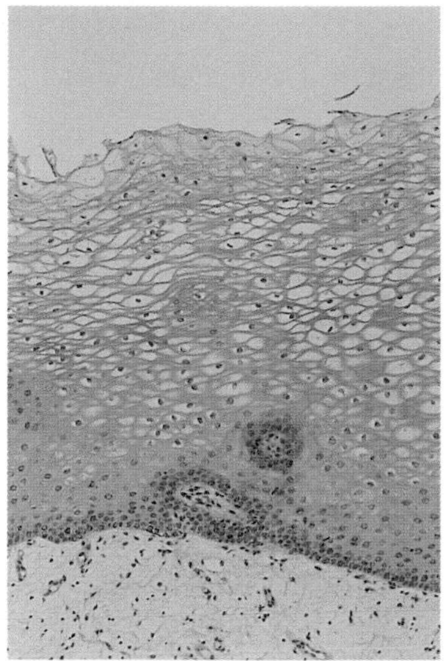

Fig. 171 Leukoedema. Vacuolation of the prickle cells.

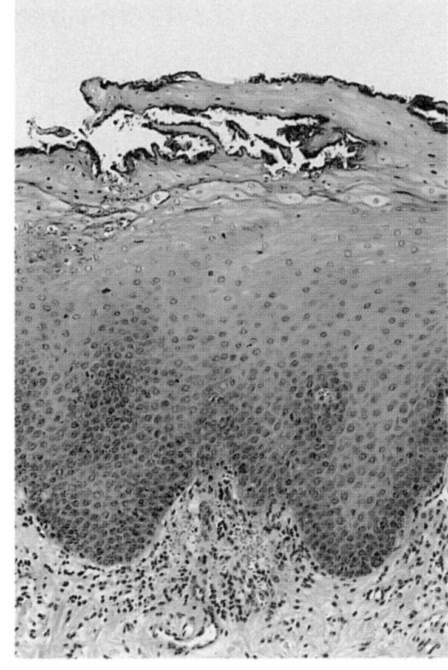

Fig. 172 Cheek-biting. Colonies of bacteria have infected the parakeratotic epithelium.

Erythema migrans

Erythema migrans (geographical tongue) appears to be an anatomical variant, though in about 5% there is an association with psoriasis. Also, there appears to be a genetic component and the abnormality may be seen in more than one member of the family or in several generations.

Clinically, children, and even very young infants, can be affected, but it seems rarely to be noticed then and most patients are middle aged. Fissuring of the tongue may be associated, and adults particularly may complain of soreness. The tongue, and rarely other mucosal sites, show irregular red areas sometimes with a conspicuous slightly raised white margin forming scalloped patterns. The characteristic feature is the change in these appearances from day to day as the areas spread or recede over the mucosa.

Microscopy

The appearances vary. Commonly, the central red areas are atrophic while the advancing margins show acanthosis, with oedema and neutrophil infiltration of the epithelium, giving an appearance similar to candidosis but without fungal hyphae. There is a variable inflammatory infiltrate in the corium (Fig. 173).

Behaviour and prognosis

Treatment is not required but reassurance may need to be given.

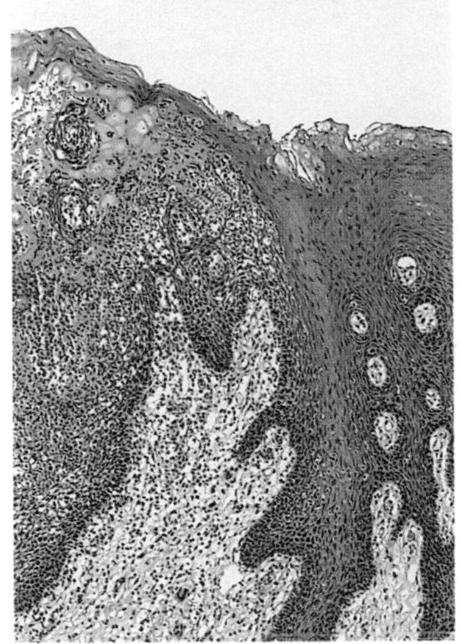

Fig. 173 Erythema migrans. Acanthotic, advancing margin.

Frictional keratosis

This shows non-specific keratosis microscopically (Fig. 174) and is distinguishable only by clinical evidence of mechanical trauma and resolution with removal of the irritant.

Prognosis

Resolution quickly follows removal of the irritant and confirms the diagnosis.

Smoker's keratosis

This results from heavy long-term pipe smoking, is therefore seen in men, and affects the palate.

Microscopy

The keratosis is non-specific but there is characteristically inflammation and swelling of the palatal mucous glands producing red umbilicated swellings (Fig. 175).

Prognosis

Prolonged pipe smoking is associated with a raised risk of cancer. However, the palatal white lesion is benign and any oral carcinoma that develops usually appears lower in the mouth such as the retromolar region.

Syphilitic leukoplakia

A feature of the tertiary stage of syphilis but rarely seen now. It typically affects the dorsum of the tongue and there is a high risk of malignant change.

Microscopy

Features of epithelial keratosis are not specific but dysplasia or malignant change may be evident (Fig. 176).

A characteristic syphilitic inflammatory response (endarteritis (Fig. 177), plasma cell infiltrate and occasionally granuloma formation) may be seen deeply, but diagnosis is essentially serological.

Prognosis

The risk of malignant change in syphilitic leukoplakia is very high.

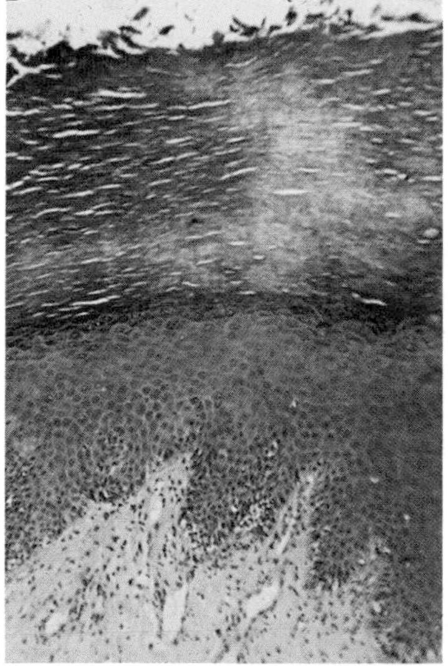

Fig. 174 Frictional keratosis.

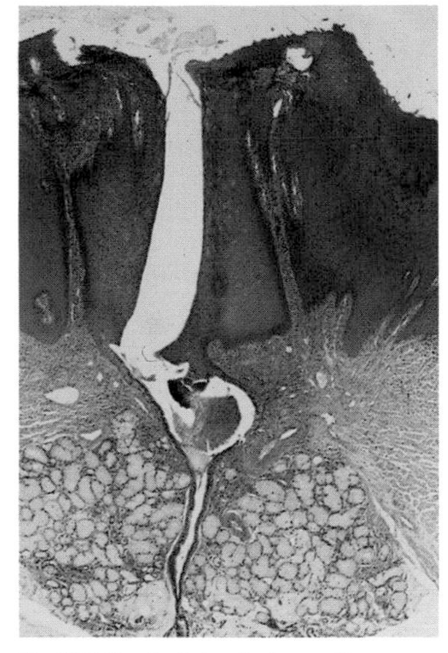

Fig. 175 Smoker's keratosis: swollen palatal salivary tissue.

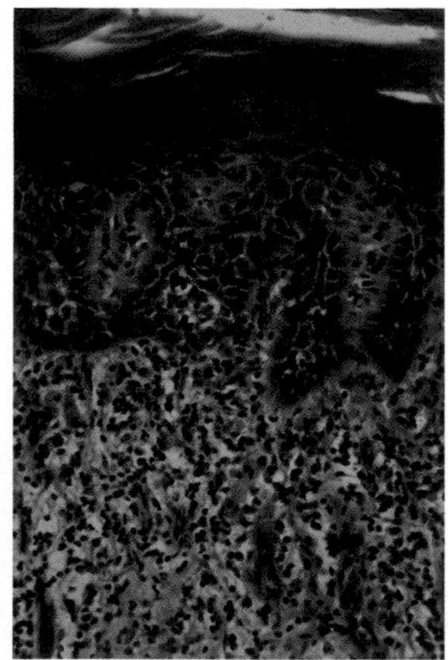

Fig. 176 Syphilitic leukoplakia with mild dysplasia.

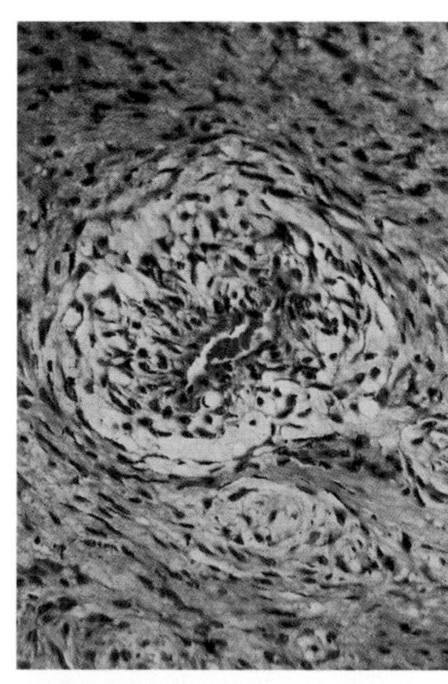

Fig. 177 Endarteritis beneath syphilitic leukoplakia.

Acute candidosis (thrush; 'pseudomembranous' candidosis)

Aetiology

Thrush is the typical acute infection of mucous membranes by *Candida albicans*. It implies underlying immunodeficiency, e.g. neonates, HIV infection, prolonged broad spectrum antimicrobial, immunosuppressive and cytotoxic treatment or debilitating illness.

Clinically, thrush forms soft friable, creamy flecks or plaques that wipe off easily revealing intact but erythematous epithelium. A Gram-stained smear shows many Gram-positive hyphae of *C. albicans* and inflammatory cells (Fig. 178).

Microscopy

The plaque of thrush is due to epithelial proliferation, i.e. it is **not** a pseudomembrane (adherent slough). The epithelial cells of the plaque are separated by inflammatory exudate (hence it is friable) including many neutrophils.

The inflammatory infiltrate is most dense, forming microabscesses, at the surface of the prickle cell layer and provides the plane of cleavage that allows the plaque to be wiped off. PAS staining demonstrates candidal hyphae growing downwards through the epithelial cells to the surface of the spinous cell layer (Fig. 180). Deeply, there is acanthosis with long, slender downgrowths of epithelium, and inflammatory cells infiltrating the lamina propria (Fig. 179).

Treatment

Thrush frequently responds well to topical antifungals such as nystatin or amphotericin but in severe immunodeficiency (e.g. HIV infection) fluconazole may be needed.

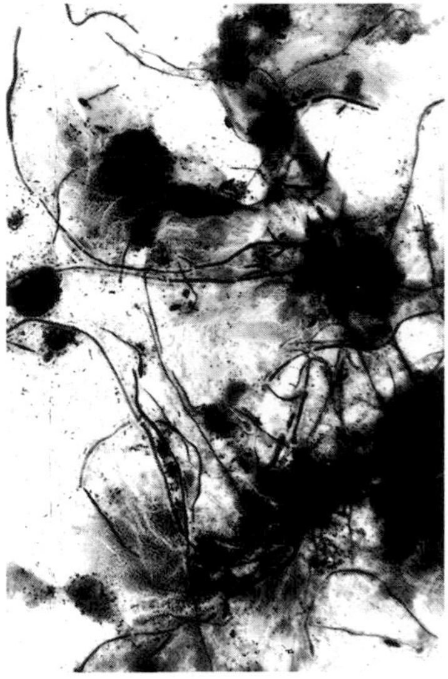

Fig. 178 Thrush: tangled hyphae in smear. (Gram stain.)

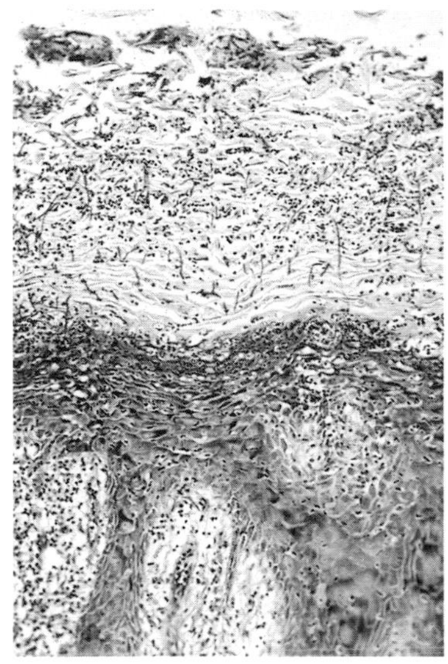

Fig. 179 Thrush: plaque. (PAS.)

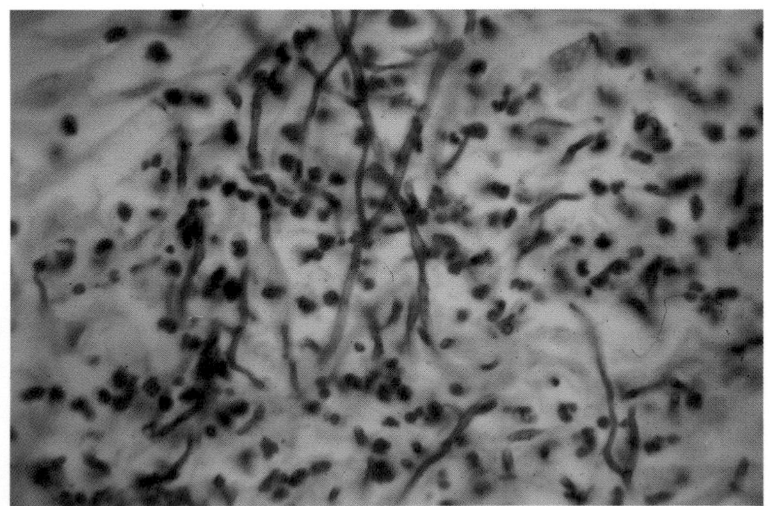

Fig. 180 Thrush: hyphae in plaque. (High power; PAS.)

Chronic hyperplastic candidosis (candidal leukoplakia)

Uncommon, persistent candidal infection usually of middle age or over but occasionally seen in patients with HIV infection, who may develop any type of oral candidosis. Clinically, chronic candidal plaques may be homogeneous or speckled.

Microscopy

Production of parakeratotic plaque. Hyphae grow through plaque to the spinous layer (Figs 181 & 182). Plaque is infiltrated by moderate numbers of leukocytes and beads of oedema. The deeper epithelium is acanthotic, sometimes grossly so (Fig. 183), and sometimes dysplastic.

Chronic mucocutaneous candidosis syndromes

All are rare but comprise leukoplakia-like oral candidosis associated with variable skin and nail involvement, and sometimes systemic disorders. There is a limited defect of cellular immunity in about 60% of patients but no special susceptibility to systemic candidosis. One variant is associated with endocrine deficiencies, particularly primary hypoparathyroidism and Addison's disease (candida endocrinopathy syndrome).

Microscopy

As for isolated chronic candidosis (see Figs 181–183).

Denture-induced erythematous candidosis

Most common under an upper denture where hyphae of *C. albicans* proliferate in the interface between denture base and mucosa, which is cut off from local defenses. Diffuse candidal erythema is also seen in xerostomia.

In HIV infection *C. albicans* can cause red mucosal macules (erythematous candidosis).

Microscopy

Hyphae are superficial to the epithelium and not seen in sections. The epithelium is spongiotic, acanthotic and infiltrated by chronic inflammatory cells.

Hairy leukoplakia

See pages 159–160.

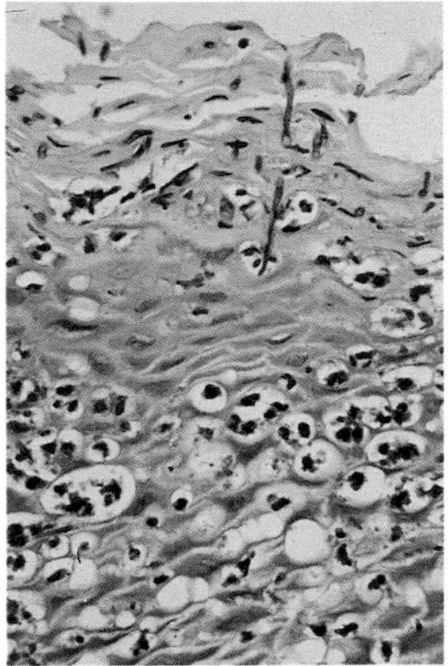

Fig. 181 Chronic candidosis: hyphae invading parakeratotic plaque. (PAS.)

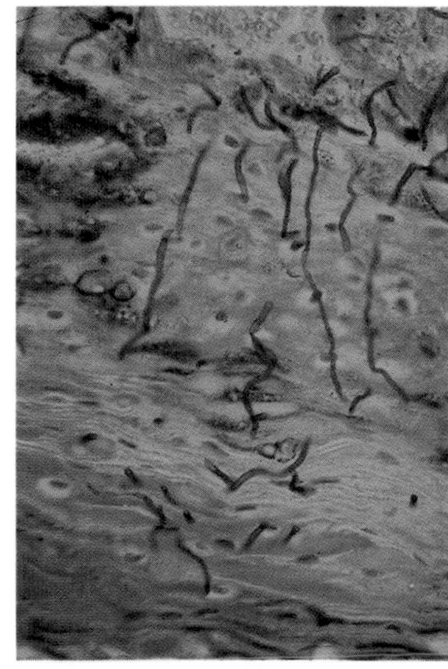

Fig. 182 Chronic candidosis: hyphae and inflammatory infiltrate in plaque.

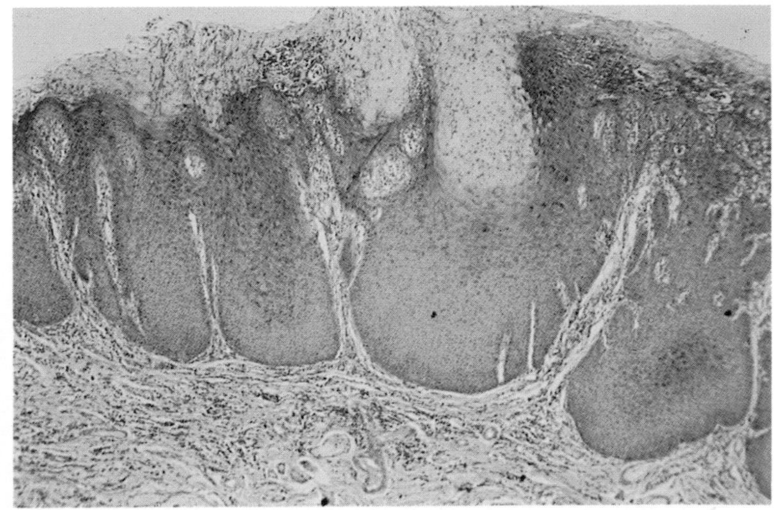

Fig. 183 Chronic candidosis: plaque and gross acanthosis.

Dysplasia (epithelial atypia; dyskeratosis)

Dysplasia is abnormal maturation and differentiation of the epithelium, as seen in carcinomas and also in some leukoplakias, when it is usually an indication of premalignancy. The following features are seen in varying combinations.

Microscopy

- Hyperchromatism and alteration of the nuclear cytoplasmic ratio. Nuclei are abnormally large in relation to the area of cytoplasm and more heavily basophilic. Nucleoli may be more prominent or numerous. Nuclear pleomorphism (irregularly shaped nuclei) is often associated (Fig. 184).
- Individual, deep cell keratinization (dyskeratosis). Individual cells within the prickle cell layer develop intracytoplasmic keratin and become eosinophilic (Fig. 185).
- Loss of polarity. The basal cell layer loses its normal orderly arrangement and the cells lie irregularly at angles to one another (Figs 185 & 186).
- Mitoses. These may be seen superficially among the spinous cells and are of sinister import, particularly if abnormal.
- Other features. Loss of intercellular adherence with fluid-filled spaces appearing between the epithelial cells (Fig. 186) and drop-shaped (bulbous) rete ridges are sometimes associated with dysplasia. Hyperkeratosis and/or acanthosis may or may not be associated.

Severe dysplasia with cellular abnormalities extending through the full thickness of the epithelium (top-to-bottom change) is sometimes termed *carcinoma-in-situ* (Fig. 187), i.e. the cellular abnormalities of carcinoma are present but there is no invasion.

Behaviour and prognosis

Dysplasia indicates a strong risk of malignant change. However, some dysplastic lesions undergo spontaneous regression and the level of risk is unpredictable even from the histological findings. The assessment of the latter is also highly subjective.

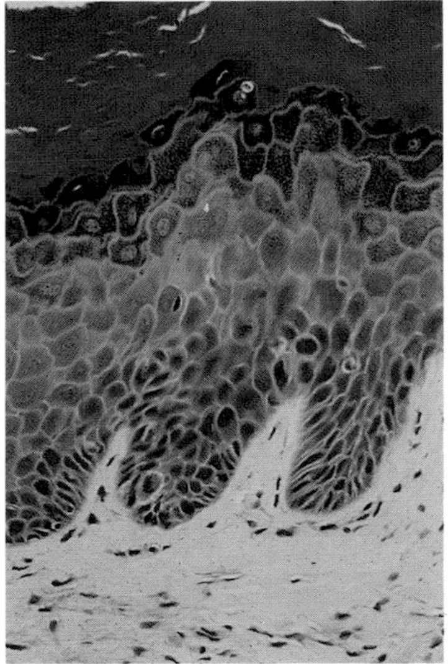

Fig. 184 Mild to moderate dysplasia with hyperchromatism and hyperkeratosis.

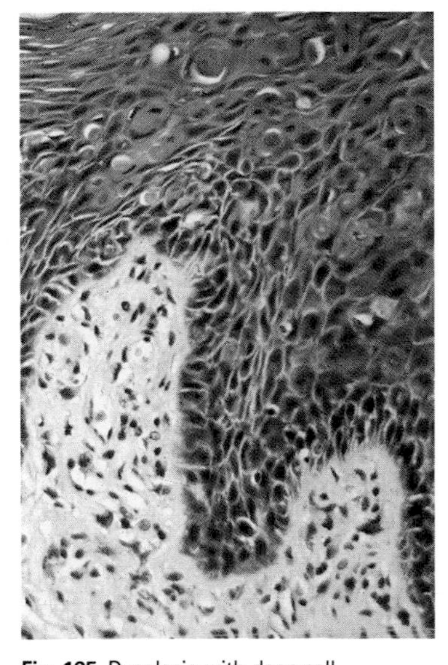

Fig. 185 Dysplasia with deep cell keratinization: hyperchromatism and loss of polarity.

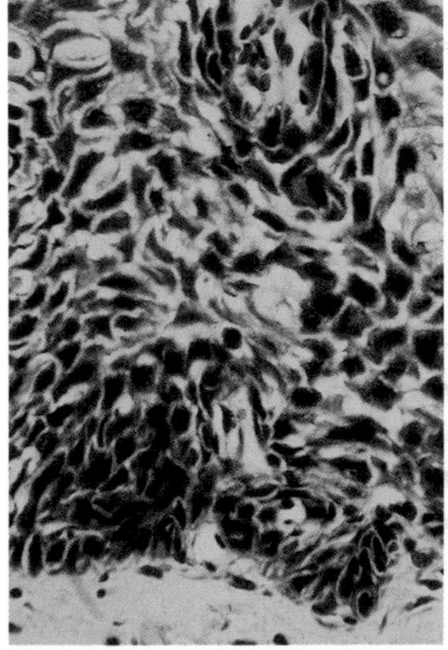

Fig. 186 Dysplasia: loss of intercellular adherence.

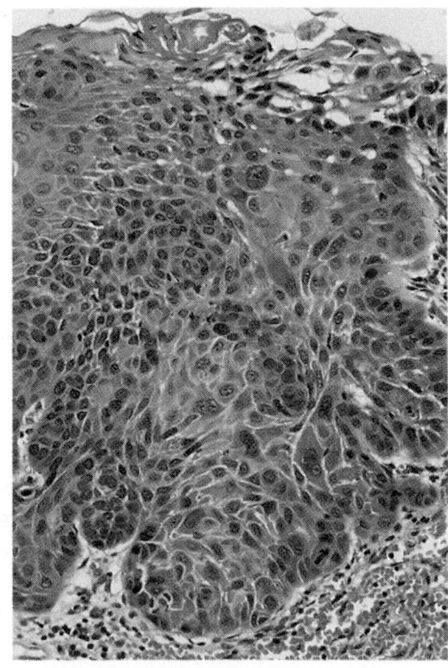

Fig. 187 Severe dysplasia (top-to-bottom change, carcinoma-in-situ).

Erythroplasia ('erythroplakia')

This is a clinical term for chronic red lesions (i.e. hyperkeratosis is absent). They do not form raised plaques but are typically level with, or depressed below, the surrounding mucosa and typically show severe dysplasia (Fig. 188) or early carcinoma.

Early keratinizing carcinoma

In addition to dysplastic leukoplakias, some early carcinomas, before ulcerating, produce keratin on the surface and appear clinically as innocent white lesions.

Microscopy

Invasive squamous cell carcinoma replaces the normal epithelial surface with an overlying parakeratinized plaque (Fig. 189).

Squamous cell papilloma

A common, benign lesion characterized by fine, finger-like papillae, giving it a warty appearance clinically. HPV (particularly types 6 and 11) may be implicated, but cytological signs of viral infection are not seen histologically. Oral viral warts resemble papillomas clinically, but show viral changes and inclusion bodies histologically.

Microscopy

A central branching core of vascular connective tissue extends into the papillae. The latter are covered by hyperplastic stratified squamous epithelium which may be keratinized (Fig. 190). The papilloma then appears white.

Treatment

Excision is curative.

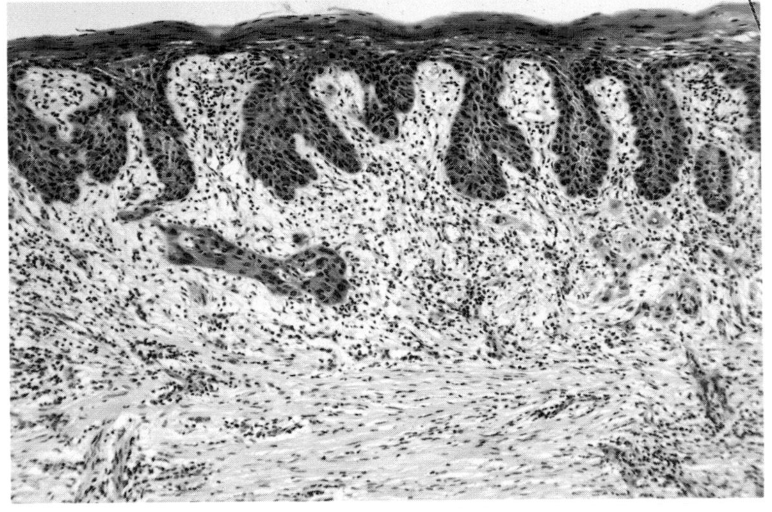

Fig. 188 Erythroplasia.

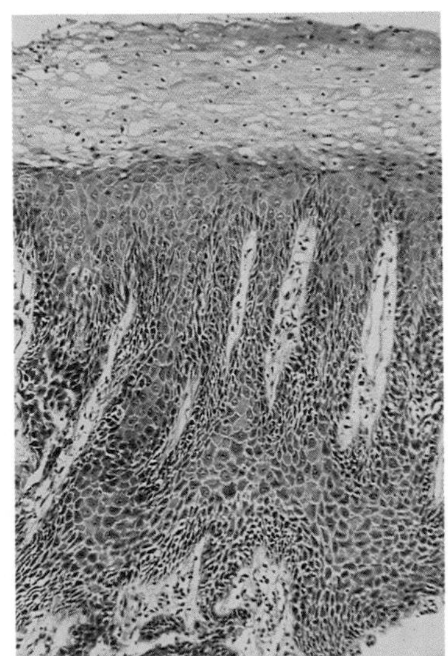

Fig. 189 Carcinoma with keratinized surface.

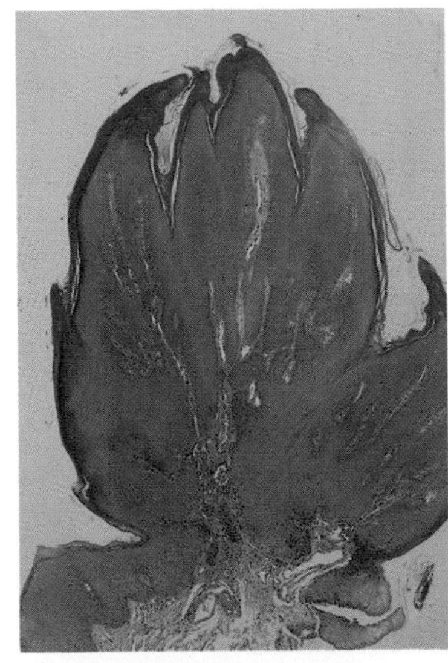

Fig. 190 Squamous cell papilloma.

14 / Squamous cell carcinoma

Aetiology and pathology

Aetiological factors usually unidentifiable although widely regarded as related to tobacco and alcohol use. There is a closer relationship with pipe than cigarette smoking. The high incidence of oral cancer in India is possibly related to different types and forms of tobacco usage. HPV 16 and related strains have been implicated, possibly by triggering inactivation of the *p53* gene. Squamous cell carcinoma usually develops after age 50 and the incidence rises with age.

Lip cancer is associated with excess exposure to sunshine, especially in fair skinned males. It is associated with leukoplakia in only a minority.

Microscopy

Essential features are epithelial abnormalities (dysplasia) and invasion. Later, metastases develop, particularly in regional lymph nodes. Most are well differentiated with obvious squamous pattern and formation of whorls of keratin deeply (cell nests) (Fig. 191).

The basement membrane tends to disappear and the tumour forms invading, irregular epithelial processes or sheets of cells with ill-defined outlines typically surrounded by chronic inflammatory cells (Fig. 192). Invasion is characterized by destruction of tissues in the path of the tumour (Fig. 193).

Neoplastic epithelial cells are pleomorphic, show variably enlarged, often hyperchromatic, nuclei or vesicular nuclei with prominent or multiple nucleoli (Fig. 194). Mitoses (see Fig. 195, p. 112) may be numerous and atypical. With increasing dedifferentiation, the neoplastic cells may become progressively more uniformly hyperchromatic and irregular in size so that they may become difficult to recognize as carcinomas by light microscopy in extreme (anaplastic) examples. Spread is primarily via lymphatics, but haematogenous spread to distal sites depends on invasion of blood vessels (see Fig. 196, p. 112). ➡

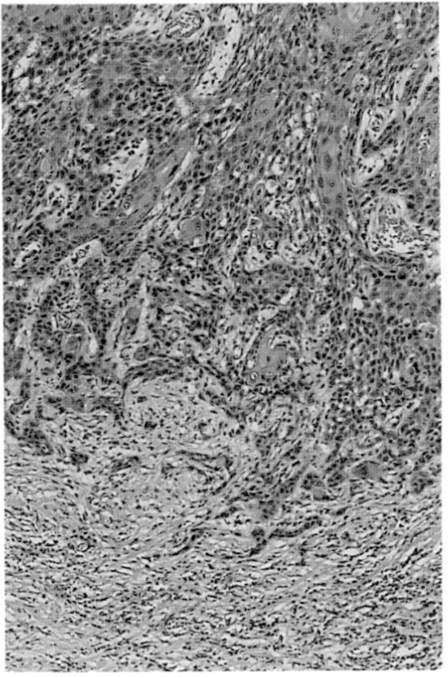

Fig. 191 Oral squamous cell carcinoma.

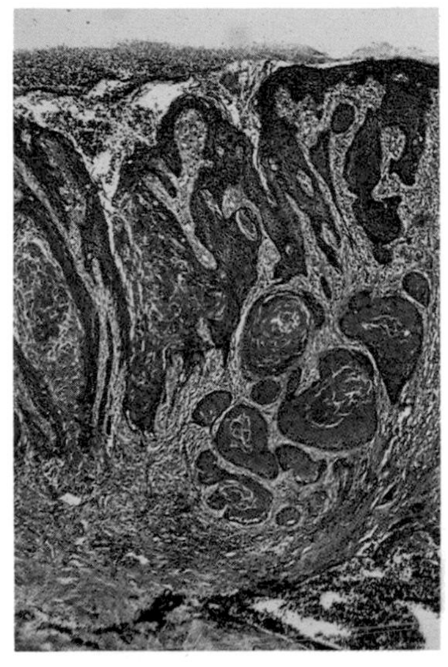

Fig. 192 Squamous cell carcinoma: well-differentiated.

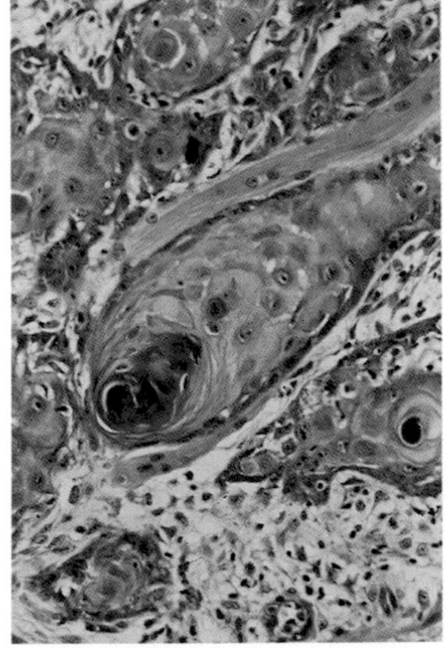

Fig. 193 Squamous carcinoma destroying muscle.

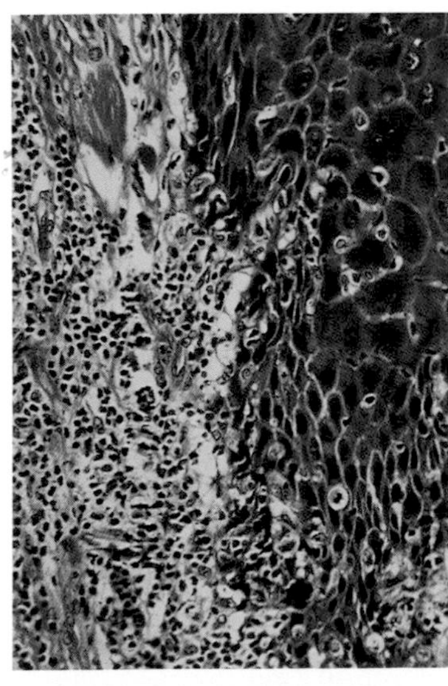

Fig. 194 Squamous carcinoma: atypia.

Treatment and prognosis

The main forms of treatment are wide excision often with radiotherapy, or radiotherapy alone. Good survival rates depend on early diagnosis and treatment. Survival also deteriorates with age. Average 5-year survival rates for carcinoma of the tongue are 37% for males and 46% for females. Most other sites within the mouth have a rather better prognosis.

Carcinoma of the lip has a much better prognosis and a 5-year survival rate of 94% for males but (inexplicably) only 84% for females.

Verrucous carcinoma

An uncommon variant which appears as a prominent white warty plaque. It may result from the prolonged use of smokeless tobacco (snuff dipping) but frequently no cause is apparent. HPV 2a–e may be implicated.

Microscopy

Gross hyperkeratosis and papillary epithelial overgrowth produces a folded appearance with intervening cleft-like spaces. The uniform level of downgrowth of the tumour gives a well-defined deep margin in the pre-invasive stage (Fig. 197), but can transform to invasive carcinoma. Epithelial atypia is minimal (in the early stages), but there is typically a chronic inflammatory infiltrate in the corium.

Treatment and prognosis

Spread and metastasis is slower than squamous cell carcinoma and the response to adequate excision is better.

Verrucous hyperplasia

An essentially similar lesion to verrucous carcinoma but differing histologically in that the mass does not push down into the lamina propria and the basement membrane zone is level with that of the surrounding normal epithelium.

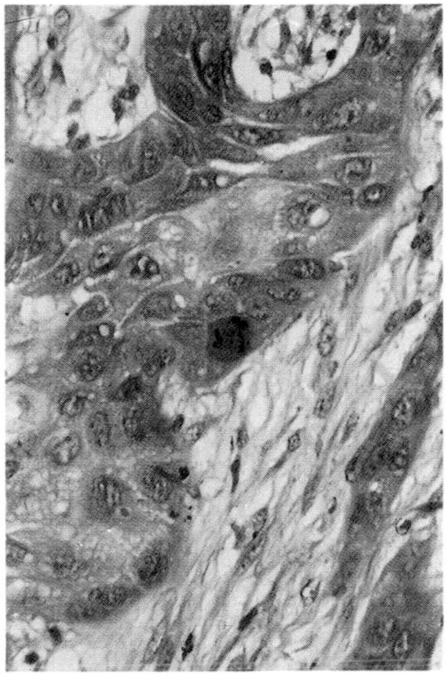

Fig. 195 Squamous carcinoma: abnormal mitoses.

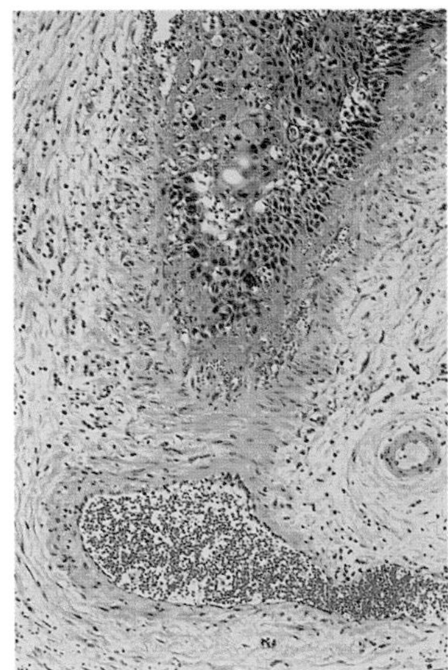

Fig. 196 Squamous cell carcinoma: tumour extending along a vein.

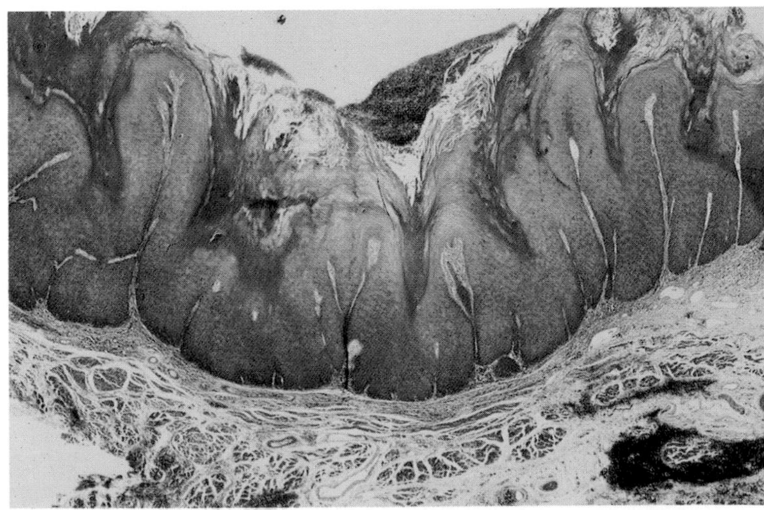

Fig. 197 Verrucous carcinoma.

15 / Hyperplastic lesions

Fibrous nodules (fibrous epulides, polyps and denture granulomas)

Aetiology and pathology

These are some of the most common oral swellings but are hyperplastic, not neoplastic, resulting from fibrous proliferation in response to chronic irritation often with an inflammatory component.

Microscopy

These lesions are distinguishable only by their site of origin and consist of irregular bundles of collagenous connective tissue with varying numbers of fibroblasts covered by stratified squamous epithelium (Figs 198–200), often with mild subepithelial inflammatory infiltrate. Osteoid or bone may form within a fibrous epulis (Fig. 201). More severe and deeply extending inflammation results from ulceration.

Treatment

Adequate excision should be curative.

Pyogenic granuloma

Clinically, pyogenic granulomas appear as soft, red nodules, usually on the gingival margins. Despite their name, these are vascular proliferations, but inflammation is frequently superimposed.

Microscopy

Many dilated thin-walled blood vessels lie in a loose connective tissue stroma but typically, inflammatory cells fill the vessels and infiltrate the stroma (see Fig. 202, p. 116). The nodule is covered by stratified squamous epithelium of variable thickness and, particularly in the inflamed type, may be ulcerated.

Treatment

Excision is curative.

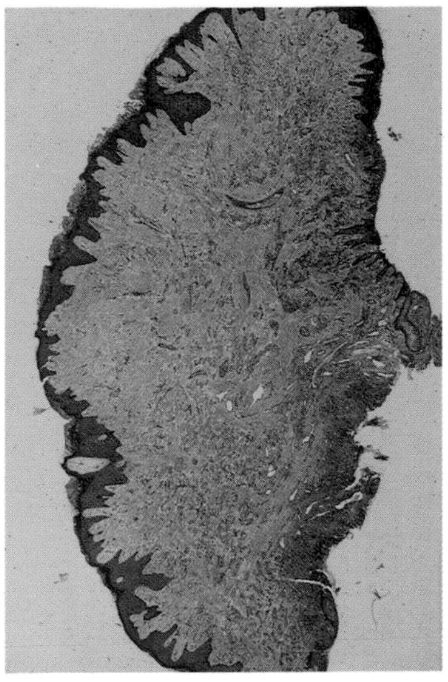

Fig. 198 Fibrous epulis.

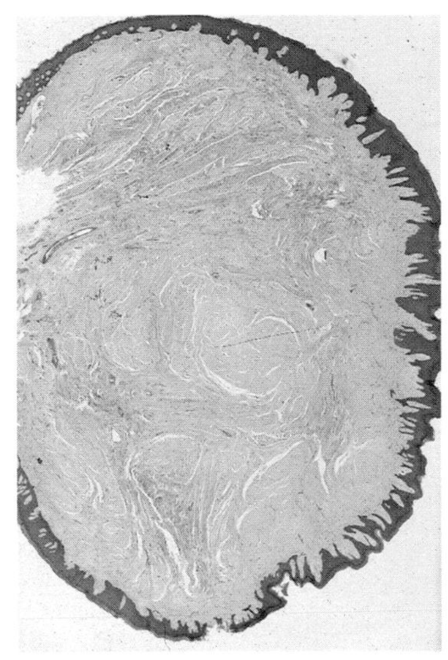

Fig. 199 Fibrous polyp of cheek.

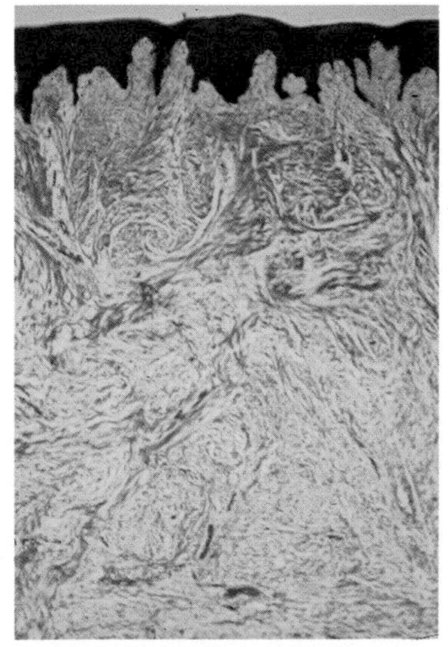

Fig. 200 Fibrous nodule: general structure.

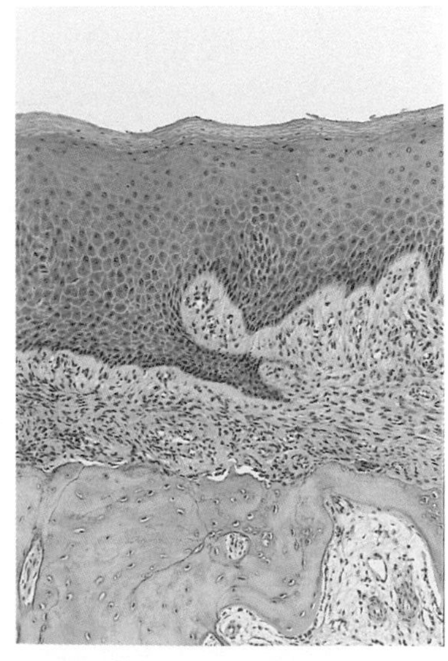

Fig. 201 Fibrous epulis with ossification.

Pregnancy epulis

During pregnancy, hormonal factors favour gingival hyperplasia and formation of pyogenic granulomas (pregnancy epulis). Clinically and histologically these do not differ from pyogenic granulomas seen in non-pregnant persons—only the pregnant state differentiates them (Fig. 203).

Treatment and prognosis

Pregnancy epulis is likely to regress after parturition if oral hygiene is good, but may have to be excised.

Giant cell epulis

This hyperplastic lesion is believed to result from a proliferation of osteoclasts from the sites of shedding of deciduous teeth as it is only found in this area of the alveolar ridge and mainly in young people. Exceptionally rarely, hyperparathyroidism gives rise to a giant cell epulis, distinguishable only by abnormal blood chemistry and bone lesions, if present.

Microscopy

The highly cellular mass is crowded with osteoclast-like giant cells of variable size in a cellular and vascular stroma and covered by stratified squamous epithelium (Figs 204 & 205). If neglected, it may undergo gradual fibrosis with a shrinking core of giant cells surrounded by fibrous tissue.

Treatment

Excision is curative.

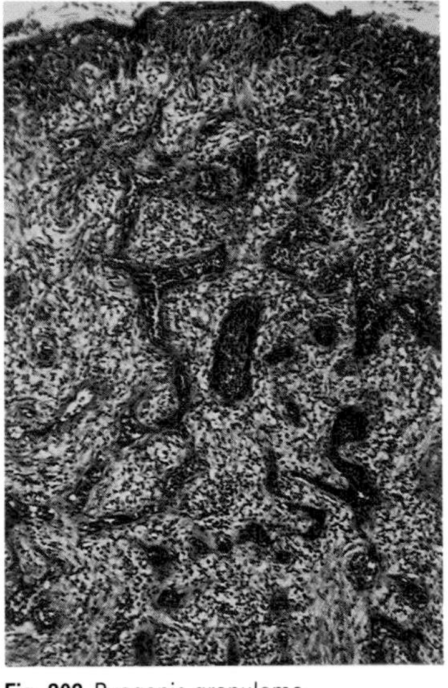

Fig. 202 Pyogenic granuloma.

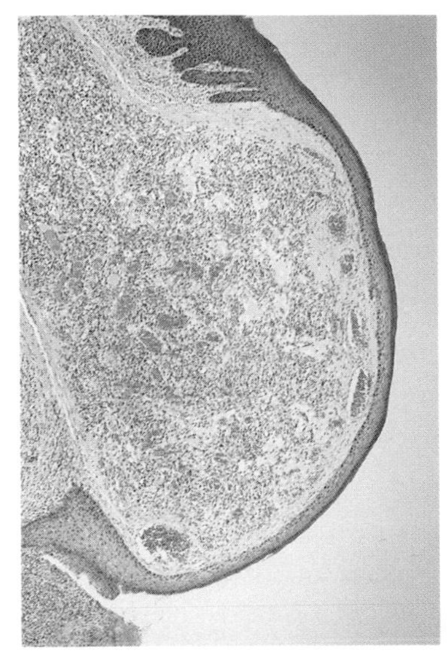

Fig. 203 Pregnancy epulis.

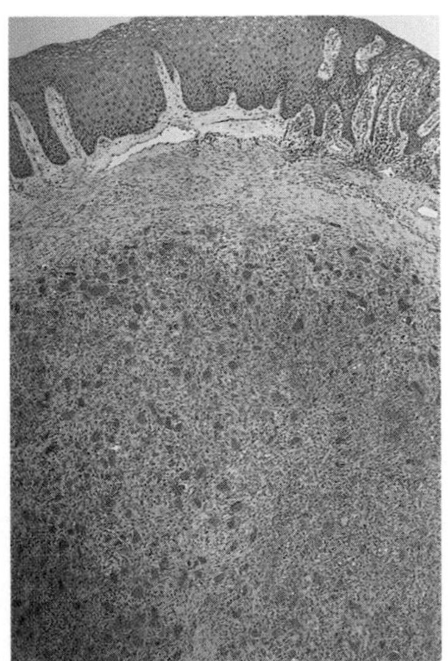

Fig. 204 Giant cell epulis.

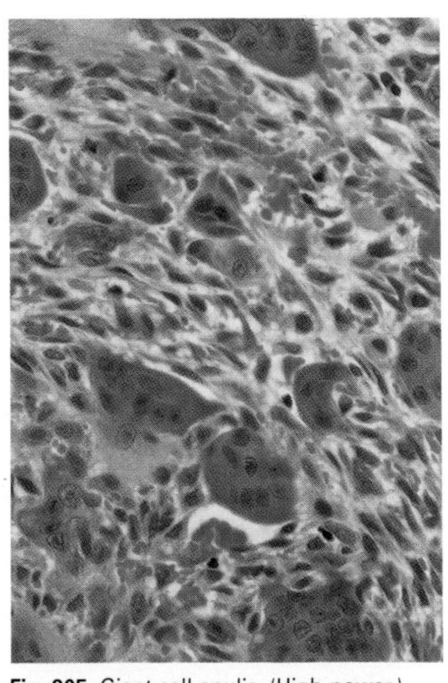

Fig. 205 Giant cell epulis. (High power.)

Neurofibroma

Neurofibromas are uncommon tumours arising from nerve sheath fibroblasts.

Microscopy

They consist of wavy bundles of collagen and fibroblasts with elongated nuclei (Fig. 206). Variable amounts of mucinous ground substance are present and may produce a myxoid appearance. The tumour may contain nerve fibres or be continuous with the sheath of a nerve.

Oral neurofibromas are rare and frequently associated with neurofibromatosis.

Neurilemmoma

Neurilemmomas arise from Schwann cells which form the axonal sheath.

Microscopy

They characteristically comprise two types of tissue:

- *Antoni A tissue*—consists of regularly arranged elongated spindle cells with closely aligned (palisaded) nuclei which are darkly basophilic and elongated (Fig. 207).
- *Antoni B areas*—consist of shorter spindle-shaped or oval cells in a mucinous matrix and wavy delicate bundles of collagen fibres.

Traumatic (amputation) neuroma

Proliferation of fibres from the proximal stump of a severed nerve can produce a tumour-like nodule of nerve fascicles surrounded by fibrous tissue (Fig. 208).

Behaviour and prognosis

Isolated neurofibromas, neurolemmonas and traumatic neuromas are benign and respond to excision.

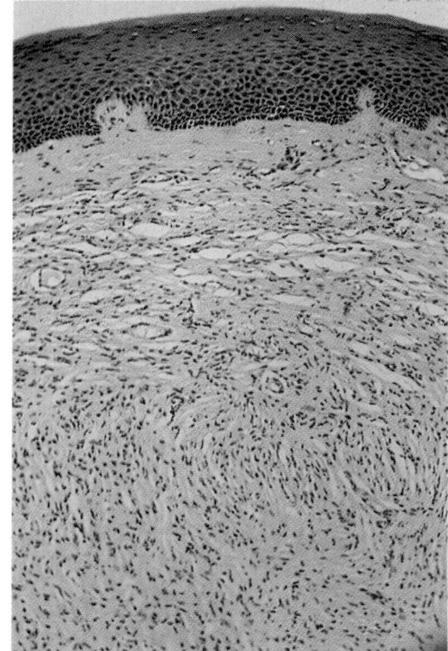

Fig. 206 Neurofibroma.

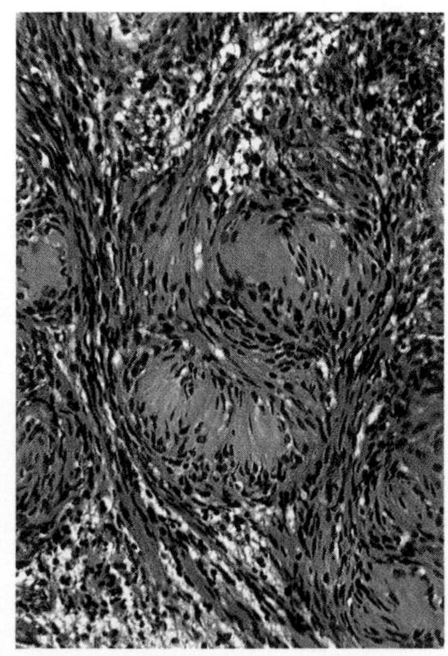

Fig. 207 Neurilemmoma.

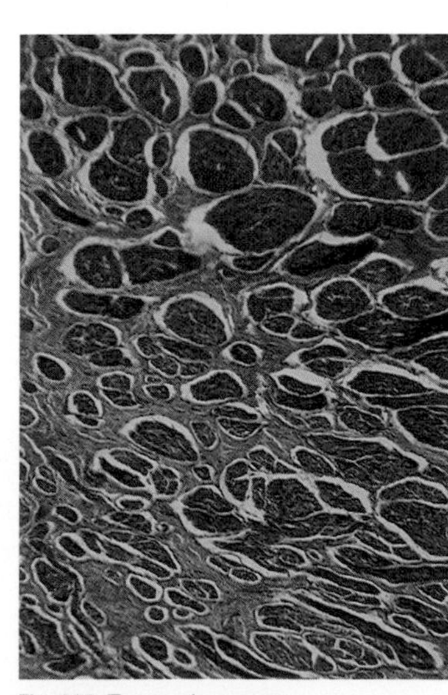

Fig. 208 Traumatic neuroma.

Plexiform neurofibroma

This consists of a tangled mass of nerve fibres cut in various planes (Fig. 209). It can be solitary but is a characteristic feature of neurofibromatosis type 1 (von Recklinghausen's disease). When found in the lateral border of the tongue, particularly, this lesion is likely to be one of the features of multiple endocrine neoplasia and associated with phaeochromocytoma and medullary carcinoma of the thyroid.

Haemangiomas

These are usually hamartomas rather than true tumours and are sometimes part of a widespread developmental defect (mucocutaneous angiomatosis, portwine stain).

Microscopy

Capillary haemangiomas
These consist of a mass of fine capillaries or imperforate rosettes of endothelial cells (Fig. 210), covered by squamous epithelium.

Cavernous haemangiomas
These consist of dilated, thin-walled, blood-filled vessels or sinusoids covered by squamous epithelium (Fig. 211). If a haemangioma needs to be removed, cryotherapy is probably then the treatment of choice because of the risk of serious haemorrhage.

Behaviour and prognosis

Soft tissue haemangiomas usually only require excision if a source of frequent bleeding secondary to trauma. Cryotherapy may lessen bleeding.

Intraosseous haemangiomas have rarely led to fatal haemorrhage when opened accidentally. Large high-flow intraosseus haemangiomas require embolization of feeder vessels before excision.

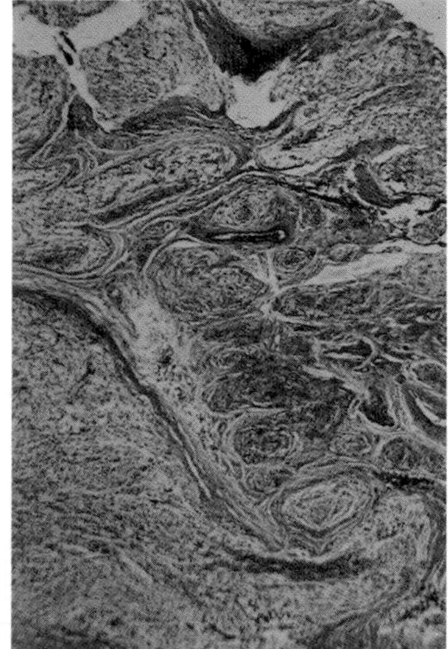

Fig. 209 Plexiform neurofibroma.

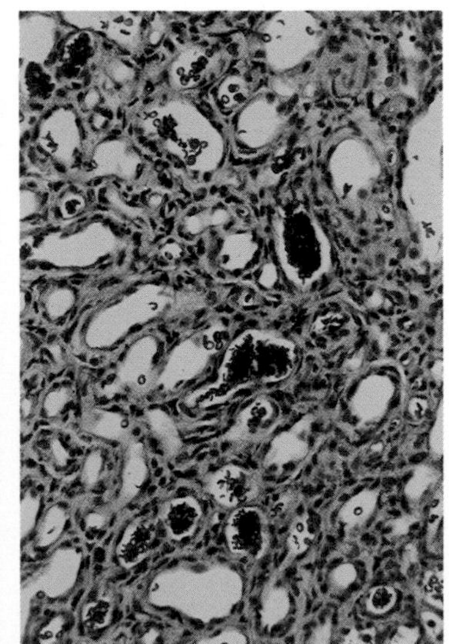

Fig. 210 Capillary haemangioma.

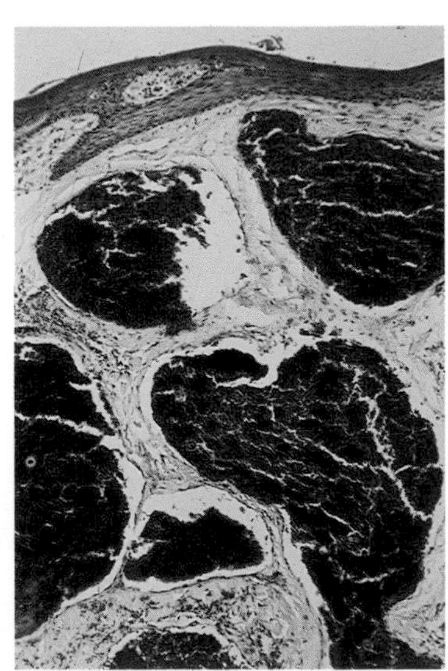

Fig. 211 Cavernous haemangioma.

Lymphangiomas

Generally resemble cavernous haemangiomas but consist of dilated lymphatic vessels which do not contain blood cells unless traumatized (Fig. 212).

Large, disfiguring lymphangiomas may require excision but this may be difficult because of the problem of defining their margins.

Vascular leiomyomas

Microscopy

These are rare, benign tumours of smooth muscle of vessel walls. They consist predominantly of smooth muscle cells which are concentrically arranged around small vessels but spread out without any regular pattern into the main tumour areas. The smooth muscle cells are not obvious in H & E stained sections but are made conspicuous with special stains such as PTAH (Fig. 213).

Leiomyomas respond to complete excision.

Lipoma

Lipomas are benign tumours of fat cells and most commonly arise from the buccal fat pad.

Microscopy

The mass consists of fat cells (adipocytes) held together by loose areolar tissue and covered by mucosa (Fig. 214).

Treatment

Excision is curative.

Liposarcomas

These are recognized but exceedingly rare oral tumours.

Wide excision is the treatment of choice but recurrence is common. The extent of the neoplasm and the histological type affect the outcome.

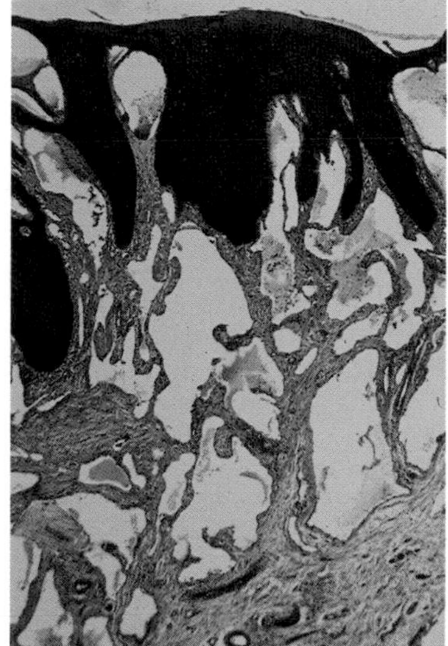

Fig. 212 Lymphangioma.

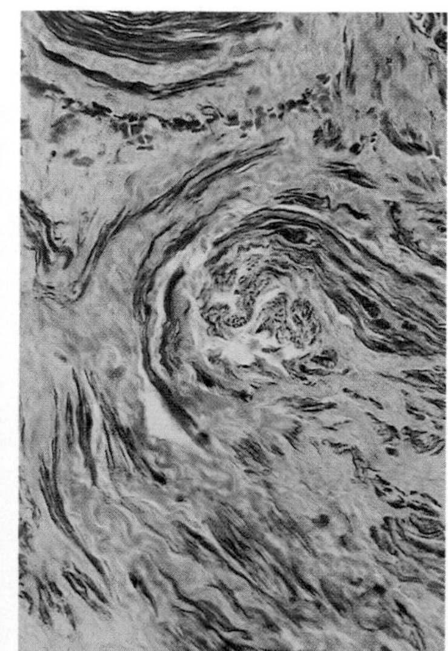

Fig. 213 Vascular leiomyoma. (PTAH stain.)

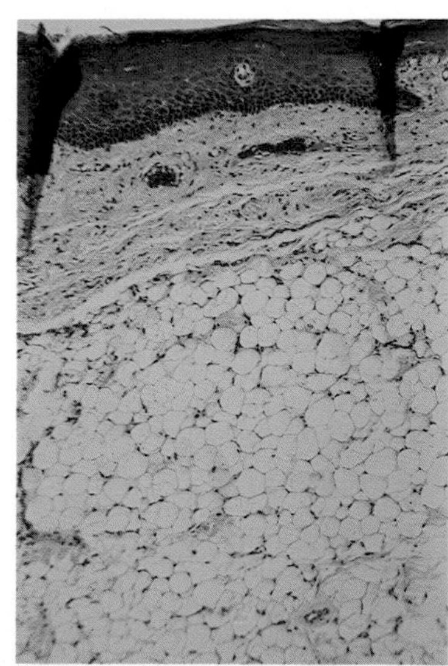

Fig. 214 Lipoma.

17 / Sarcomas

Kaposi's sarcoma

Aetiology and pathology

As a result of the worldwide spread of HIV infection, the previously rare Kaposi's sarcoma has become one of the most common types of sarcoma and is the most common oral tumour in AIDS. In HIV infection, Kaposi's sarcoma is most frequent in male homosexuals. It can also complicate deep immunosuppression but mainly in those who are HLA B5. In these conditions, Kaposi's sarcoma frequently appears in the mouth as a purplish plaque or nodule.

The tumour is thought to be of viral origin, probably HHV8, and secondary to the immunodeficiency state.

Microscopy

Kaposi's sarcoma is a tumour of endothelial cells (as shown by the marker for factor VIII) but these largely assume a spindle shape (Fig. 215). Early lesions consist of proliferating capillaries, usually with many inflammatory cells, and closely resemble granulation tissue.

Later there are fibrosarcoma-like interlacing bands of spindle-shaped tumour cells surrounding slit-like vessel lumens or minute round lumens when cut in cross-section (Fig. 216). The inflammatory element progressively disappears, the tumour cells become more pleomorphic and mitoses become numerous (Fig. 217). Interspersed are haemangioma-like areas with more obvious vascular spaces.

Prognosis

Kaposi's sarcoma has a poor prognosis in AIDS and is usually fatal within 2 years of diagnosis, if treatment fails. However, associated infections secondary to the immunodeficiency are more frequently the cause of death.

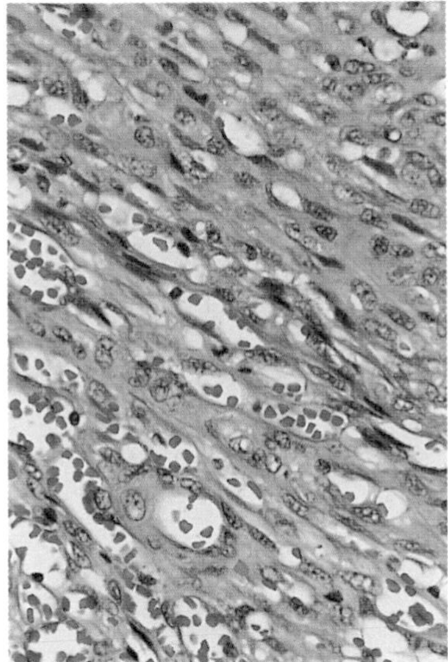

Fig. 215 Kaposi's sarcoma: proliferating endothelial cells and slit-like vascular spaces.

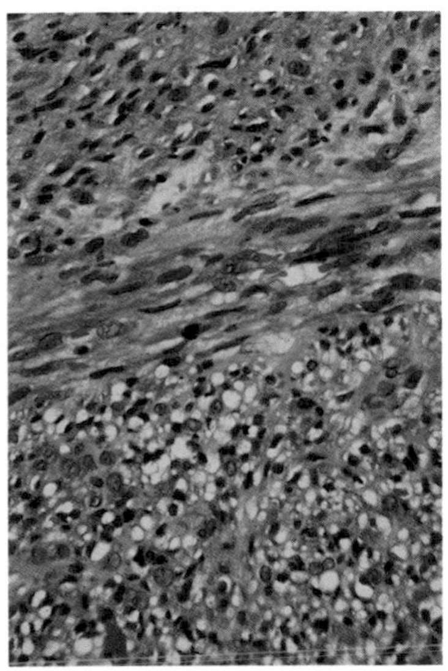

Fig. 216 Kaposi's sarcoma: spindle cells and transversely cut vascular spaces.

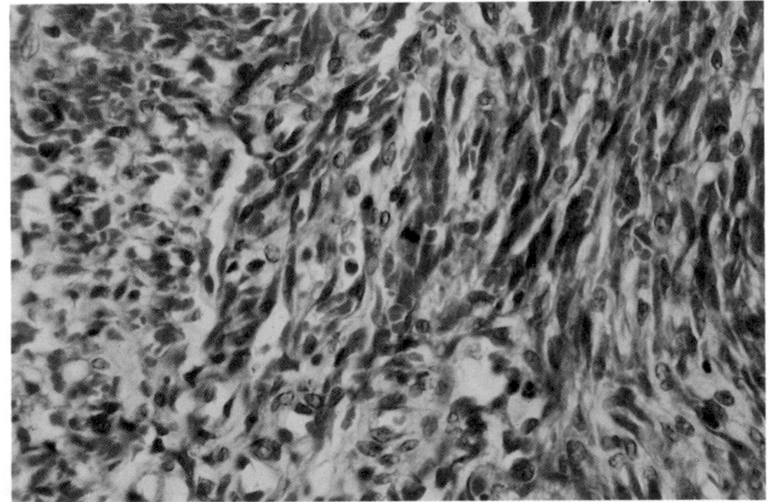

Fig. 217 Kaposi's sarcoma: mitotic activity.

Fibrosarcoma

Oral fibrosarcomas are exceptionally rare. The peak age incidence is between 35 and 55. They form firm swellings without distinctive clinical features.

Microscopy

Malignant fibroblasts form dense interlacing bundles of uniform, elongated, spindle-shaped cells with occasional mitoses and some collagen formation. With increasing dedifferentiation the arrangement of the cells becomes more irregular, mitoses become more frequent and less collagen is produced (Fig. 218). Metastases may develop many years after diagnosis and usually form in the lungs.

Rhabdomyosarcoma

Rhabdomyosarcomas are also rare but the most common type of oral sarcoma in children.

Microscopy

The alveolar type shows spindle-shaped spaces from the walls of which hang round or pear-shaped, darkly staining cells (Fig. 219).

Embryonal rhabdomyosarcomas are highly pleomorphic and consist of a loose, unorganized mass of cells without obviously identifiable features (Fig. 220) unless cross-striations are seen; immunocytochemistry for muscle cell markers is helpful.

Prognosis

Rhabdomyosarcomas are highly malignant. Radical excision followed by radiotherapy and/or chemotherapy is the usual treatment but there is frequently local recurrence or distant metastases. The lungs or bones are the main sites of metastases but lymph nodes may be involved in about 50%: death may follow in 1–6 years.

Rhabdomyoma

The main site for this rare tumour is the tongue.

Microscopy

Large, round, granular eosinophilic cells contain large amounts of glycogen and, frequently, fat spaces. Cross-striations may be seen (Fig. 221) or may be demonstrable only by special stains.

Rhabdomyomas are benign.

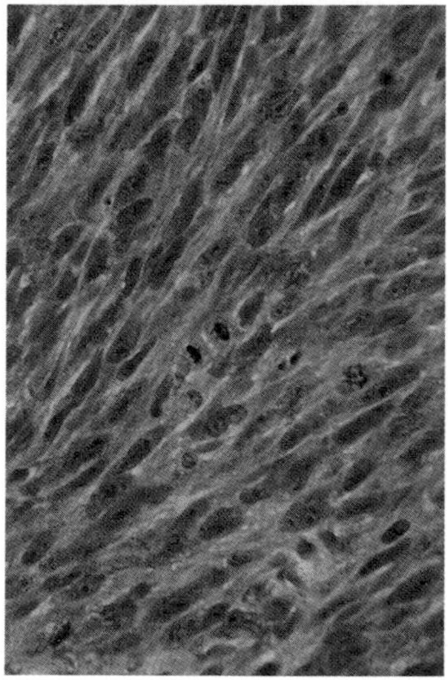

Fig. 218 Fibrosarcoma.

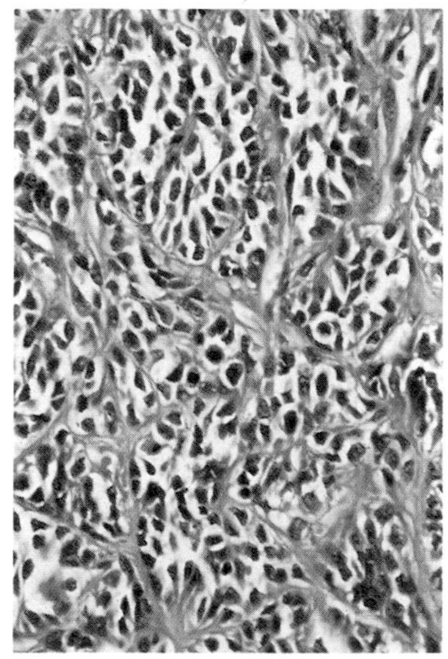

Fig. 219 Rhabdomyosarcoma: alveolar cell type.

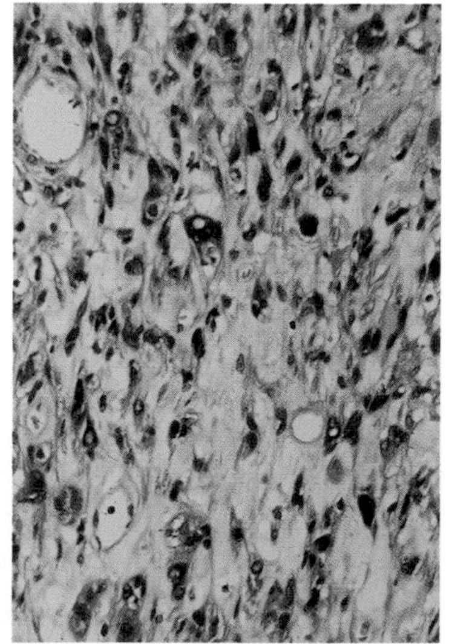

Fig. 220 Rhabdomyosarcoma: pleomorphic type.

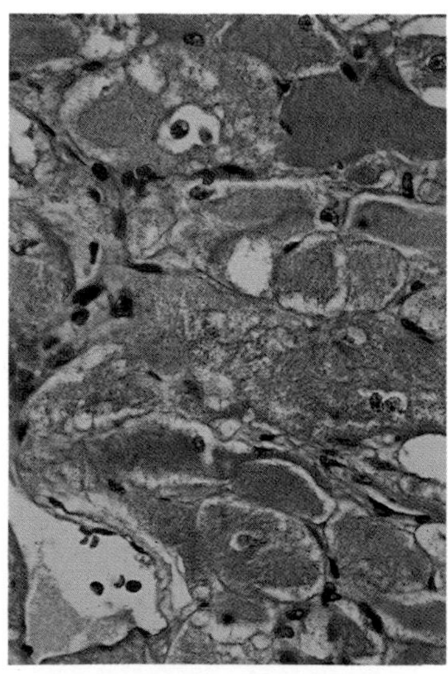

Fig. 221 Rhabdomyoma of tongue.

18 / Lymphomas

Lymphomas comprise Hodgkin's disease and non-Hodgkin's lymphoma. Non-Hodgkin's lymphoma usually arises from B lymphocytes and the different variants result from the stage of development of the lymphocyte undergoing neoplastic change. The cell of origin of Hodgkin's disease is uncertain but may be the monocyte or T lymphocyte.

Lymphomas (particularly Hodgkin's disease) are rare in the mouth, far more commonly affecting cervical lymph nodes, but are considerably more frequently seen in patients with AIDS. In the mouth they may be the primary lesion or the presenting feature of disseminated disease.

Microscopy

Lymphomas are one of the most difficult areas of histopathology, as reflected by the many classifications. The essential feature is proliferation of lymphocytes either diffusely (Fig. 222) or with a follicular pattern. According to the type, the lymphocytes range from large immature lymphoblasts to small mature cells or immunoblasts (Fig. 224). Monoclonal immunoglobulin production may be detected. Surrounding tissues may be invaded (Fig. 223). Hodgkin's disease is remarkable for the variety of cells present, including lymphocytes, histiocytes, eosinophils and Reed–Sternberg cells. The latter are large cells with a symmetrical (mirror-image) pair of large vesiculated nuclei.

Treatment and prognosis

The prognosis of non-Hodgkin's lymphoma varies according to the histological type and particularly to the stage of development when detected. If reasonably localized, Hodgkin's disease responds to radiotherapy and/or chemotherapy.

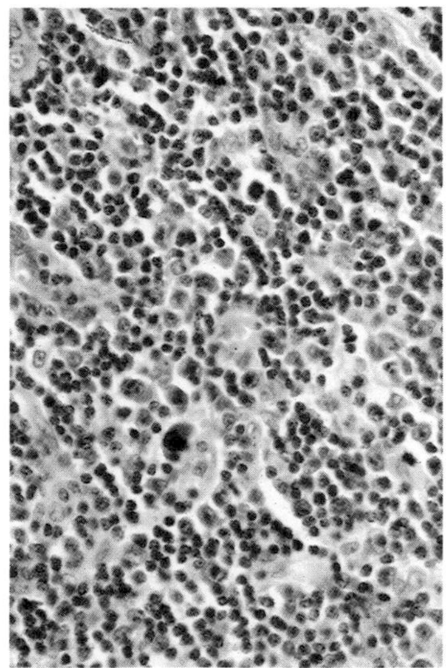

Fig. 222 Lymphocytic lymphoma.

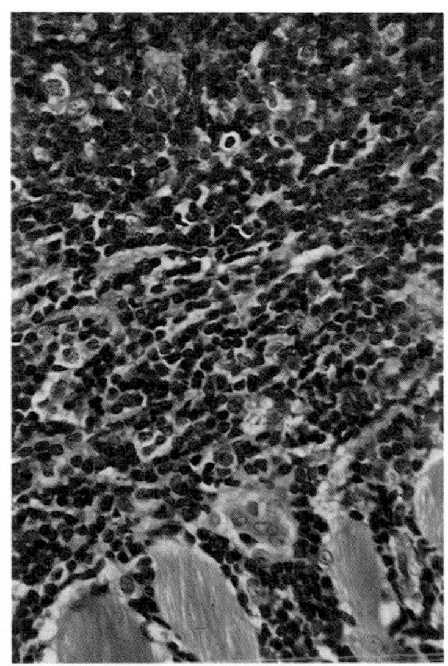

Fig. 223 Lymphoma invading muscle.

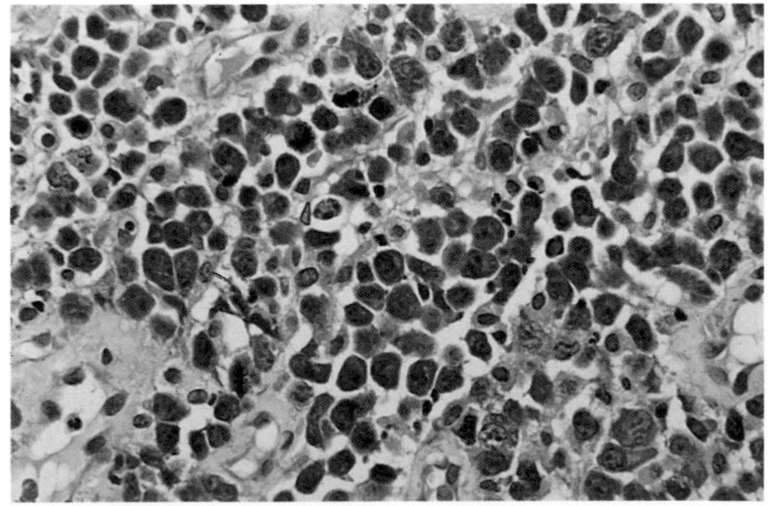

Fig. 224 Immunoblastic lymphoma.

19 / Pigmented lesions

Pigmented naevi

These range from bluish-brown macules resembling amalgam tattoos to extensive black areas, usually on the palate.

Microscopy

The pigment cells (melanocytes) can be intradermal (in the submucosal connective tissue) (Fig. 225), or junctional (clusters of melanocytes projecting from the epitheliomesenchymal junction into the underlying corium) (Fig. 226), appearing to drop down from the epithelium. In adults junctional activity is suggestive of malignant melanoma. Compound naevi show a combination of both features.

Naevi are benign but all oral pigmented lesions should undergo excision biopsy to exclude malignant melanoma.

Malignant melanoma

Oral malignant melanomas are rare, are often large before being noticed and the prognosis is therefore poor. Amelanotic melanomas appear as reddish areas or nodules. Peak incidence is at 40–60 years.

Microscopy

The features can include:

- intraepithelial melanocytes, typically with clear halos round them
- junctional activity with melanocytes in large, clear areas within and dropping from the basal layer
- proliferation of melanocytes in the submucosal connective tissue.

Malignant melanocytes range from round to spindle-shaped and can be in solid sheets, rounded, circumscribed groups or in fascicles (Fig. 227 and Figs 228–229, p. 132). Pigment may be dense or invisible without special staining.

Prognosis

Wide excision followed by radiotherapy is the usual treatment but the 5-year survival rate of oral melanomas is only about 25%.

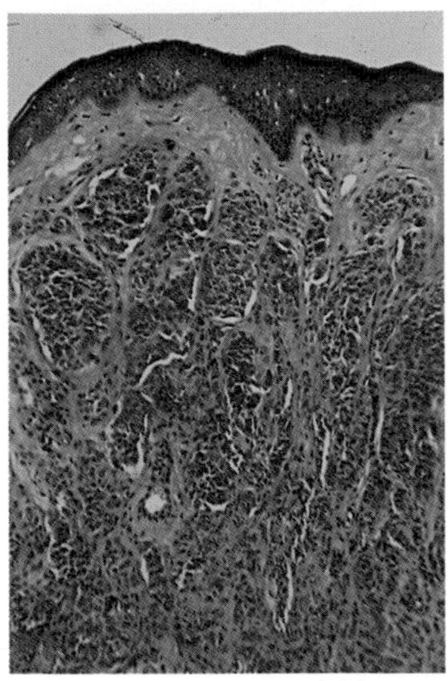

Fig. 225 Melanocytic naevus.

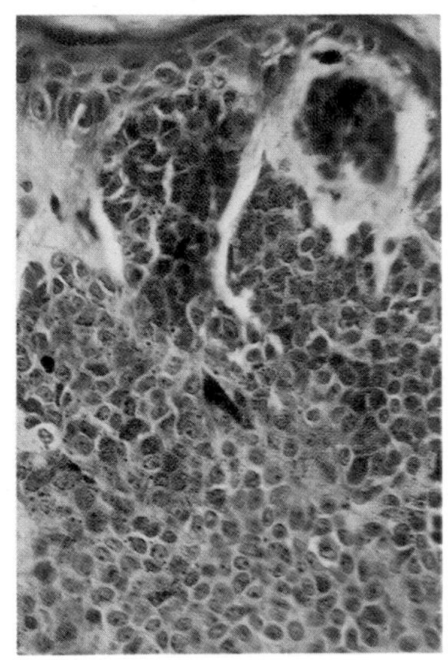

Fig. 226 Junctional activity and pigmentation.

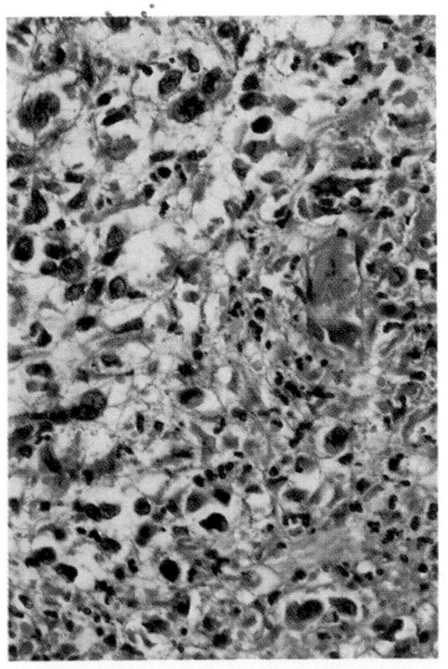

Fig. 227 Malignant melanoma: pigmented melanocytes.

Amalgam tattoo

Clinically, amalgam tattoos are by far the most common oral pigmented lesions. Histologically, the amalgam is seen as black particles or larger masses lying in the connective tissue, frequently with no foreign body reaction (Fig. 230). Biopsy is usually required to exclude an early melanoma.

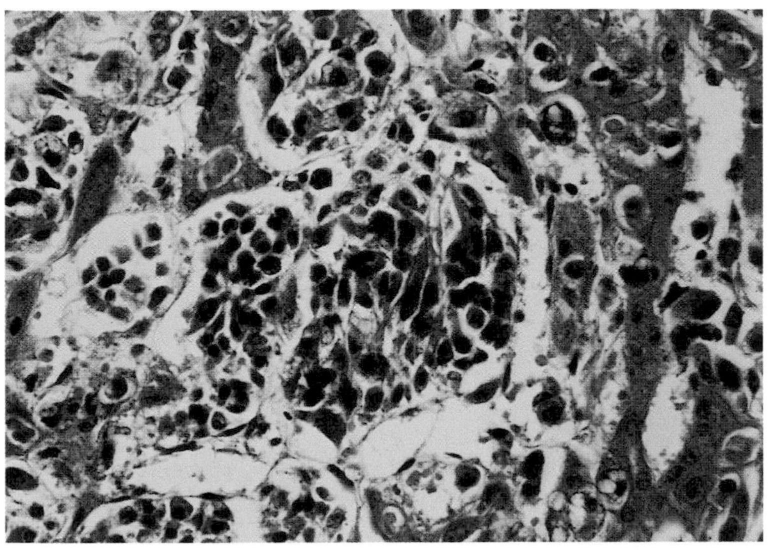

Fig. 228 Melanoma. Predominantly spindle-shaped melanocytes with variable pigmentation.

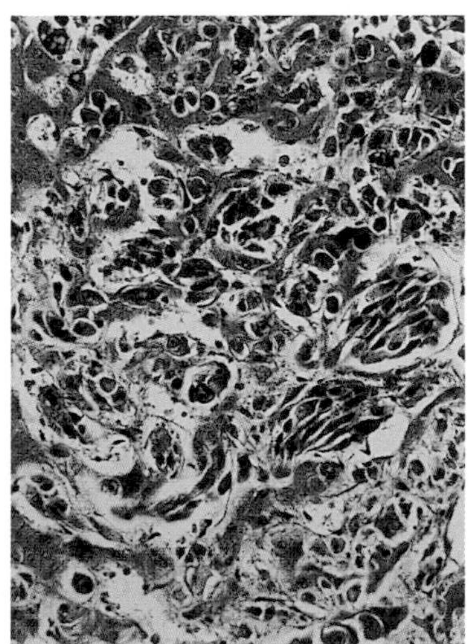

Fig. 229 Melanoma. Spindle-shaped and rounded, heavily pigmented, neoplastic melanocytes.

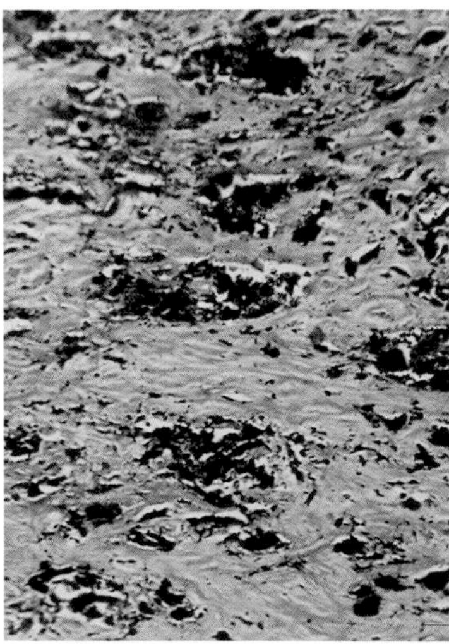

Fig. 230 Amalgam tattoo.

20 / Miscellaneous tumour-like lesions

Granular cell tumour

Clinical appearances are variable; the tumour is usually seen on the dorsum of the tongue. Adults between the ages of 30–60 years are affected.

Microscopy

Two characteristic features are:
- pseudoepitheliomatous hyperplasia of the overlying epithelium (Fig. 231)
- granular cells replacing muscle fibres (Figs 232 & 233).

The epithelium may closely resemble carcinoma but lacks cellular atypia. Cells with coarse eosinophilic granules appear to merge with muscle fibres. Positive staining for S-100 protein and neurone specific enolase suggest a neural origin.

Prognosis

Granular cell tumours are benign and respond to excision.

Granular cell epulis of the newborn (congenital epulis)

This soft, rounded swelling may rarely be found on the alveolar ridge of neonates. The upper jaw is usually affected and most are in female infants.

Microscopy

Close-packed granular cells have prominent cell membranes. The granular cells stain with myogenic markers (e.g. myosin and actin) but not for S-100 protein. The overlying epithelium is flat and lacks pseudoepitheliomatous hyperplasia.

Prognosis

The granular cell epulis is benign and responds to excision.

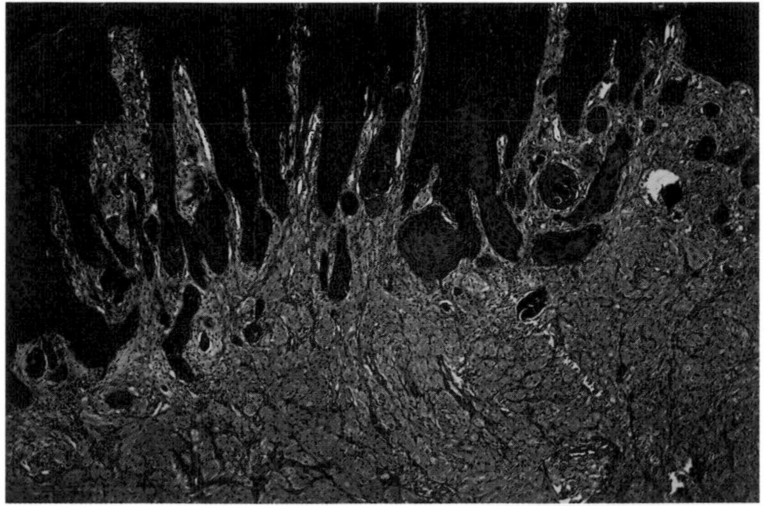

Fig. 231 Granular cell tumour: pseudo-epitheliomatous hyperplasia.

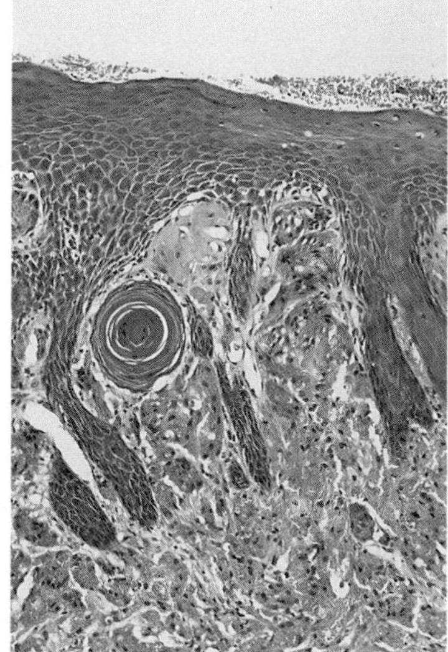

Fig. 232 Granular cell tumour: pseudoepitheliomatous hyperplasia with cell nests and granular tumour cells beneath.

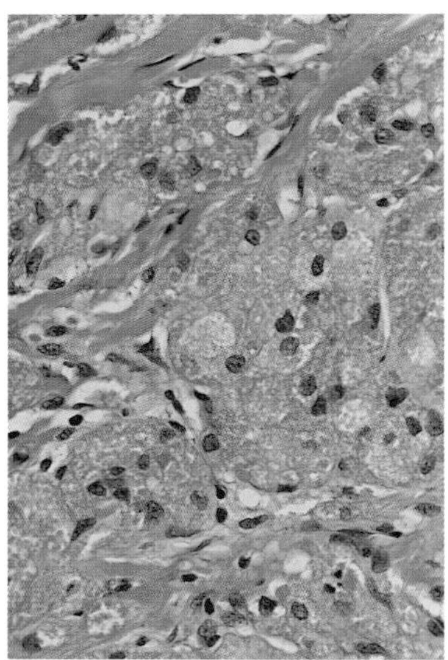

Fig. 233 Granular cell tumour: granular tumour cells merging with muscle fibres.

Pleomorphic adenoma

This is the most common type of salivary neoplasm but forms only about 40% of intra-oral salivary gland tumours. Typical intraoral sites are palate, lip and buccal glands.

Microscopy

Pleomorphic adenomas form from epithelial and myoepithelial cells. Myoepithelial cells cannot be reliably recognized by light microscopy but appear as spindle-shaped, hyaline (plasmacytoid) or clear cells. They can be identified by immunostaining positively with both epithelial and muscle cell markers. Myoepithelial cells produce the connective tissue structures in pleomorphic adenomas as a result of their multipotential properties.

Highly variable patterns are seen even within individual tumours (Fig. 234). Common features include:

- duct-like structures (Fig. 235)
- sheets of small, dark epithelial cells
- squamous metaplasia and keratin formation (Fig. 236)
- basophilic mucoid areas, sometimes forming the bulk of the tumour (Fig. 237)
- cartilage (see Fig. 238, p. 138) and, occasionally, bone
- fibroblast-like myoepithelial spindle cells
- 'plasmacytoid' hyaline myoepithelial cells (see Fig. 239, p. 138). ➡

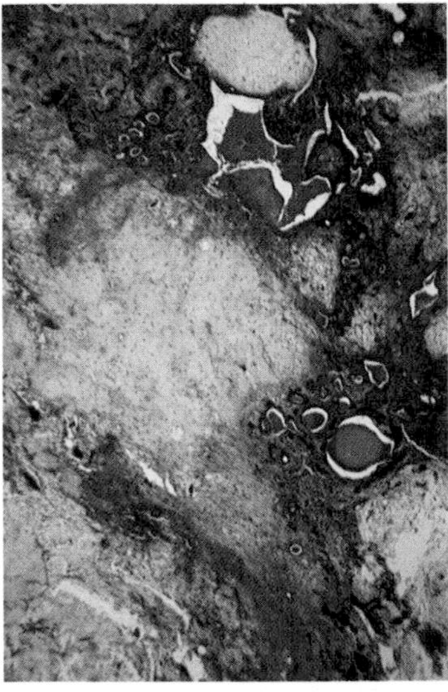

Fig. 234 Pleomorphic adenoma: typical mixed pattern.

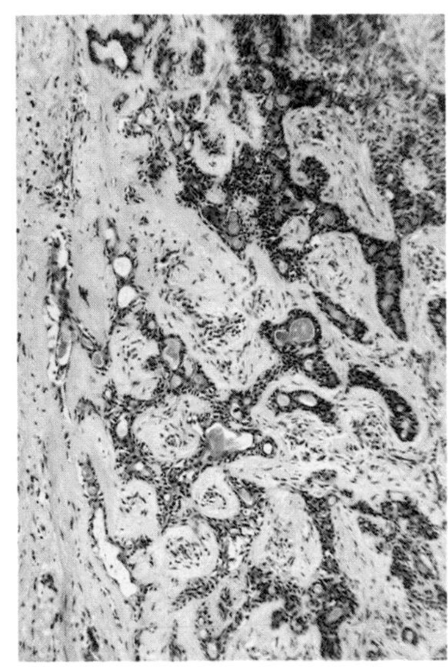

Fig. 235 Pleomorphic adenoma: tubular structures.

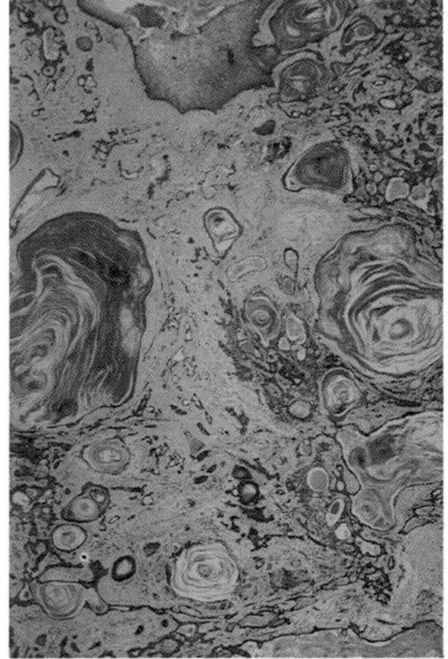

Fig. 236 Pleomorphic adenoma: squamous metaplasia.

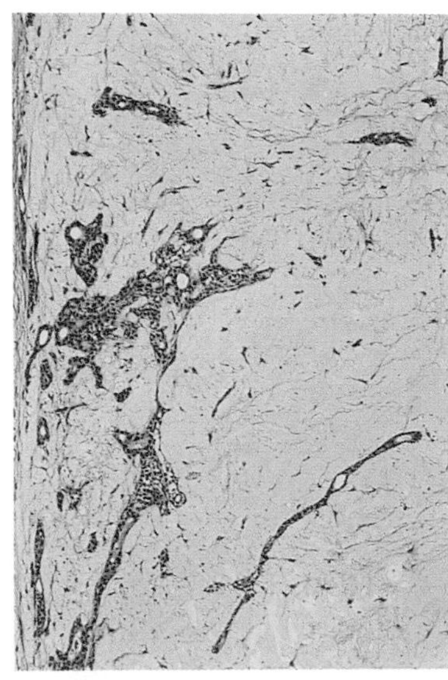

Fig. 237 Pleomorphic adenoma: myxoid type.

Pleomorphic adenoma (2)

There is a fibrous capsule, but it is frequently incomplete and tumour often extends through the capsule without invading surrounding tissues (Fig. 240).

Prognosis

Pleomorphic adenoma is slow-growing and benign but can undergo malignant change (see p. 143; Carcinoma in pleomorphic adenoma), usually after many years. Carcinoma may then be seen adjacent to typical pleomorphic adenoma components in the same tumour.

Treatment

Complete excision is essential and curative. Incomplete excision typically leads to multinodular growth and increased risk of malignant change. Recurrence of pleomorphic adenomas results from:

- surgical difficulties of removal, especially from the parotid gland
- extension of the tumour through the capsule
- seeding of spilt tumour cells into the incision (due to attempted enucleation), leading to multinodular recurrences (Fig. 241). Pleomorphic adenomas are *not* initially multinodular.

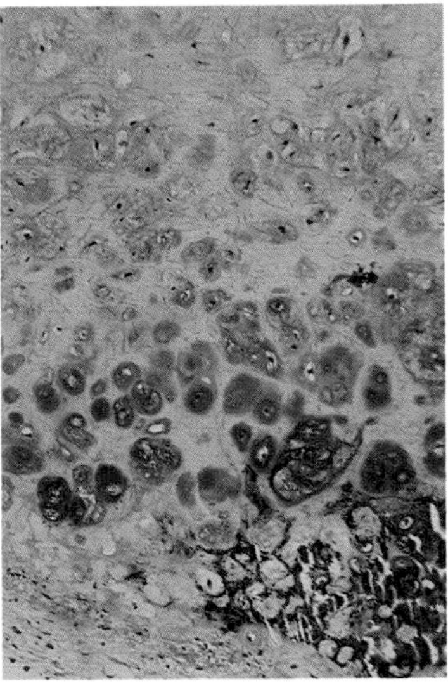

Fig. 238 Pleomorphic adenoma: cartilage with calcification.

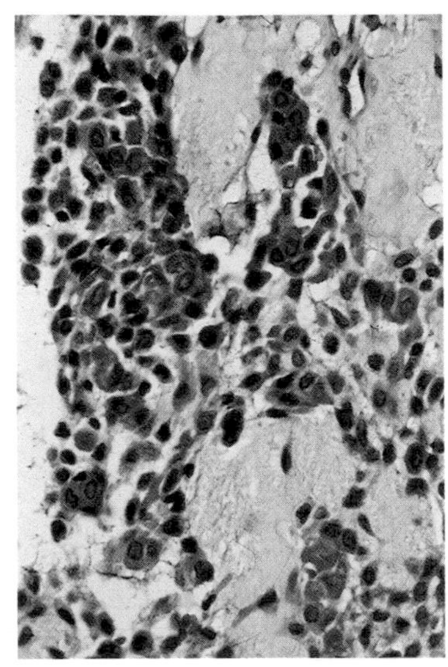

Fig. 239 Pleomorphic adenoma: hyaline cells.

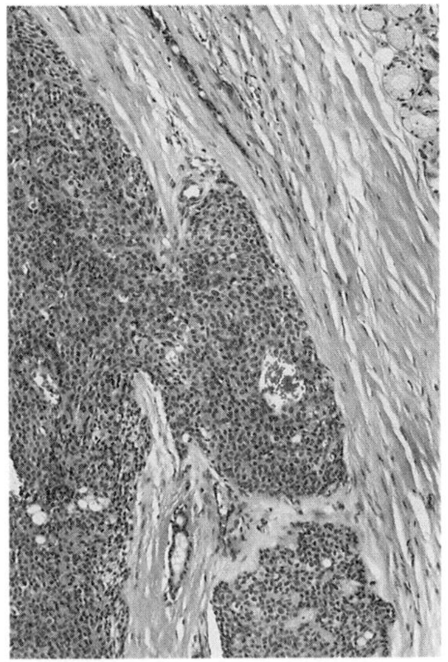

Fig. 240 Pleomorphic adenoma: infiltrating the capsule.

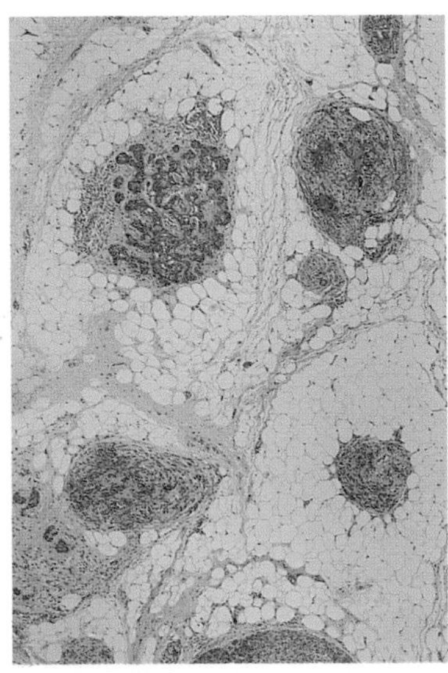

Fig. 241 Pleomorphic adenoma: seedlings from failed enucleation.

Monomorphic adenomas

These have a uniform pattern often of trabecular or canalicular pattern (Figs 242 & 243) and lack the connective tissue components of pleomorphic adenoma. There are several subtypes.

Warthin's tumour (Adenolymphoma)

Warthin's tumours form about 10% of salivary gland tumours but virtually all are in the parotid gland and about 5% are bilateral. Intra-oral glands are probably never affected. This tumour is mostly seen in middle age and typically forms a soft or cyst-like mass in the lower pole of the parotid.

Microscopy

The two components are glandular epithelium and lymphoid tissue (Fig. 244). Tall, columnar, eosinophilic epithelial cells (Fig. 245) surround and protrude into cystic spaces and cover lymphoid tissue consisting of small lymphocytes and, usually, germinal centres. The tumour is benign.

Prognosis

Monomorphic adenomas, including Warthin's tumour, are benign and have less tendency to recur after excision than pleomorphic adenomas.

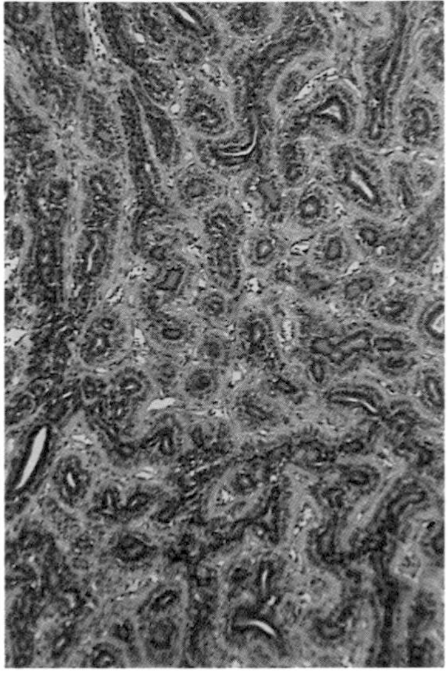

Fig. 242 Monomorphic adenoma.

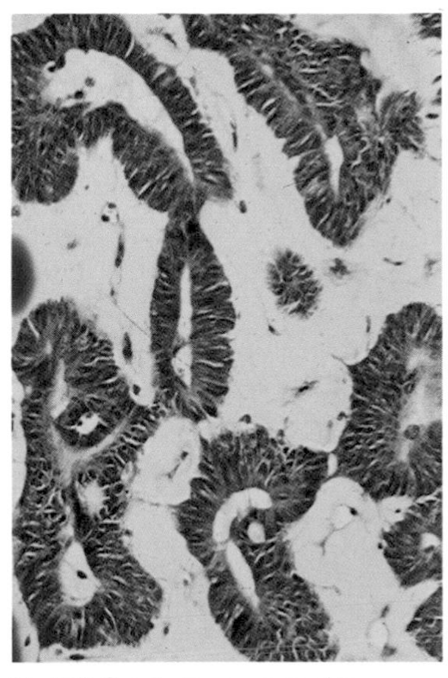

Fig. 243 Canalicular monomorphic adenoma of lip.

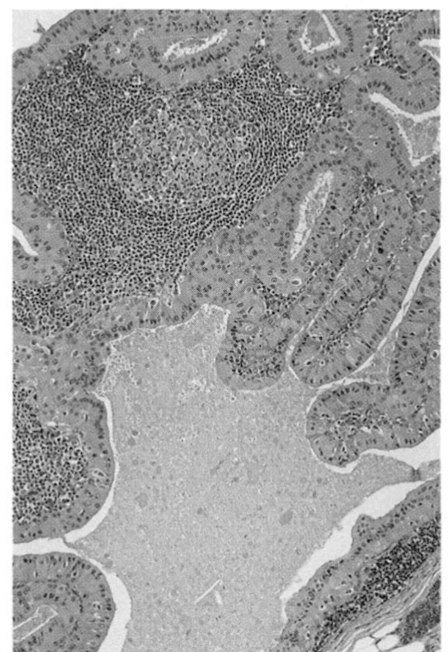

Fig. 244 Warthin's tumour.

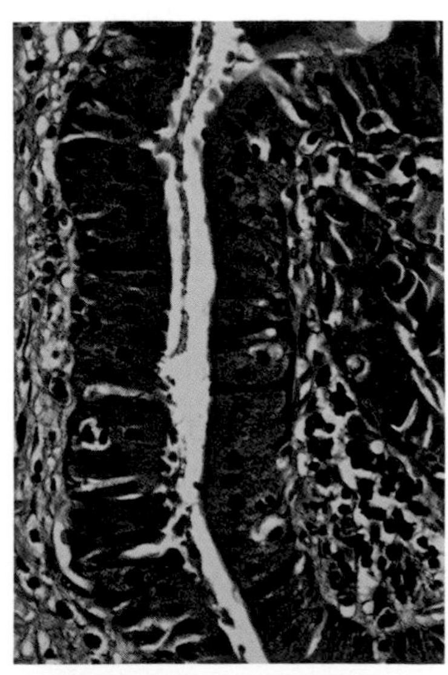

Fig. 245 Warthin's tumour: epithelial component.

Mucoepidermoid carcinoma

Mucoepidermoid carcinoma can be relatively benign or can behave like a typical carcinoma. It forms nearly 10% of intra-oral salivary gland tumours; most commonly on the palate. Patients are usually middle-aged or older.

Microscopy

The two components are large, pale, mucus-secreting cells, which typically surround large or small cystic spaces (Figs 246 & 247), and sheets of epidermoid cells. Less well differentiated tumours tend to resemble squamous cell carcinomas but for the presence of occasional mucous cells (Fig. 248).

Prognosis

Behaviour of mucoepidermoid carcinomas is not reliably predictable from histological appearances. They can be invasive and metastasize even when cytologically benign (Fig. 247). Wide excision is therefore required.

Acinic cell carcinoma

Forms only about 2% of intra-oral salivary gland tumours.

Microscopy

Typically a more or less uniform pattern of large, darkly basophilic cells with granular cytoplasm (Fig. 249) resembling serous acinar cells. Often tumour cells are in sheets without obvious organization but occasionally in an acinar arrangement.

Prognosis

Acinic cell carcinomas even when cytologically benign can also be invasive and metastasize. Wide excision is therefore required.

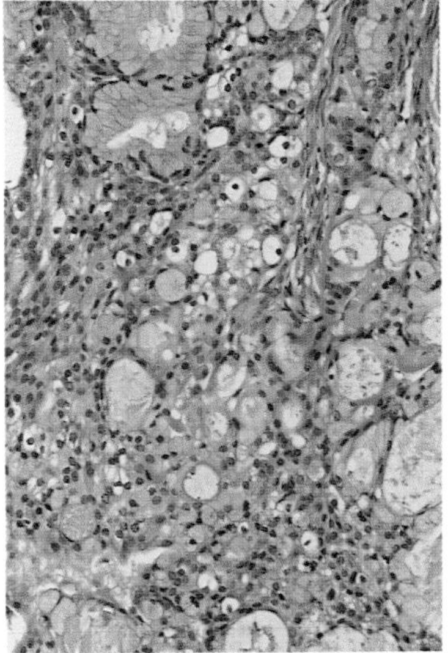

Fig. 246 Mucoepidermoid carcinoma.

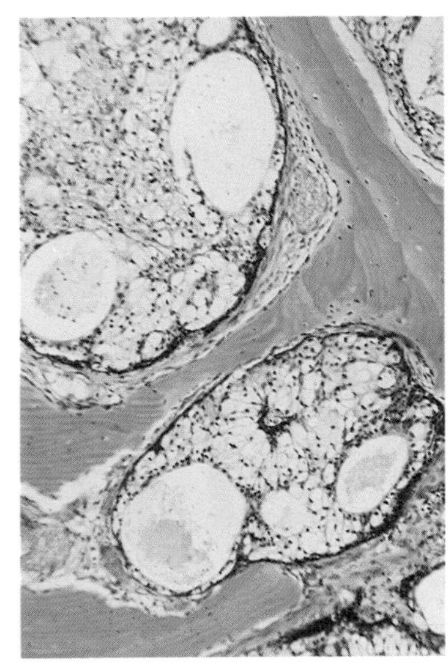

Fig. 247 Mucoepidermoid carcinoma invading bone.

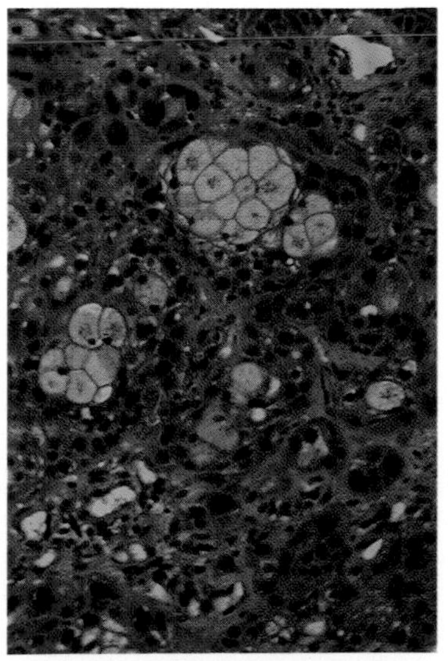

Fig. 248 Mucoepidermoid carcinoma: epidermoid and mucous cells.

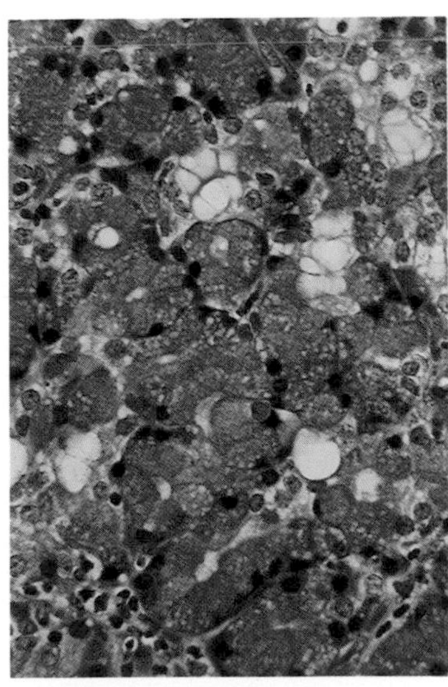

Fig. 249 Acinic cell carcinoma.

Adenoid cystic carcinoma

Forms 13% of intra-oral salivary gland tumours.

Microscopy

Typically consists of small, dark cells with duct-like 'holes' in a cribriform (Swiss cheese) (Fig. 250) or lace-like pattern, often with hyaline or mucinous change in the stroma. It has a strong tendency to perineural invasion (Fig. 251) and spread.

The tumour is slow-growing but difficult to excise as the borders are ill-defined. Metastases develop late and radical excision is needed.

Adenocarcinoma and other carcinomas

Form about 12% of intra-oral salivary gland tumours, and mainly affect the over 60s.

Microscopy

Well-differentiated tumours form glandular patterns (Fig. 252) or cysts with papillary ingrowths. Less-well-differentiated tumours show greater cellular pleomorphism.

Undifferentiated carcinomas and squamous cell carcinomas are rare and seen mostly in the elderly.

Carcinoma in pleomorphic adenoma

Pleomorphic adenoma can undergo malignant change, usually after years of slow growth, in recurrences and in old fibrotic (scarred) tumours (Fig. 253). Carcinoma in pleomorphic adenoma comprises about 7% of salivary tumours of minor glands but up to 30% of sublingual gland tumours.

Microscopy

Malignant change is usually adenocarcinoma (Fig. 253) or undifferentiated carcinoma with invasion and destruction of surrounding structures, but elsewhere features of original pleomorphic adenoma persist.

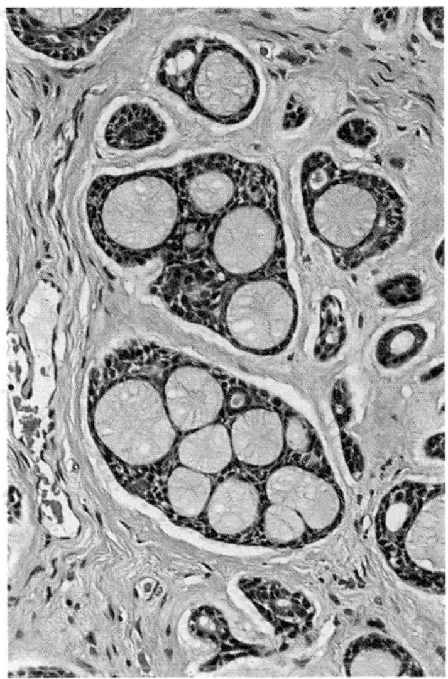

Fig. 250 Adenoid cystic carcinoma.

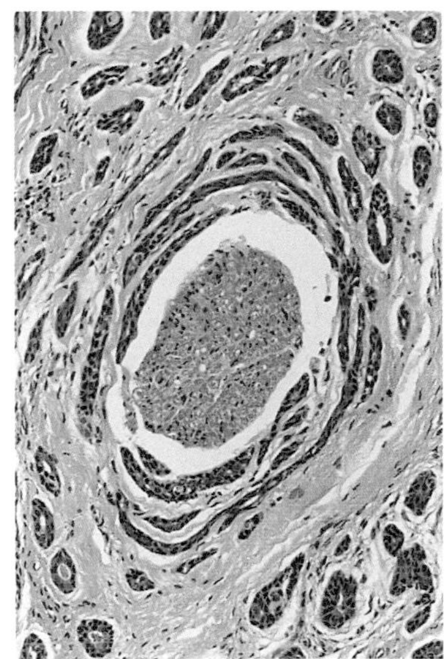

Fig. 251 Adenoid cystic carcinoma: perineural invasion.

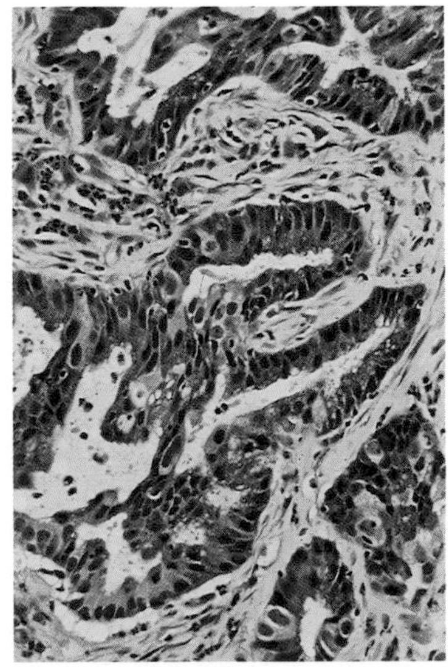

Fig. 252 Adenocarcinoma.

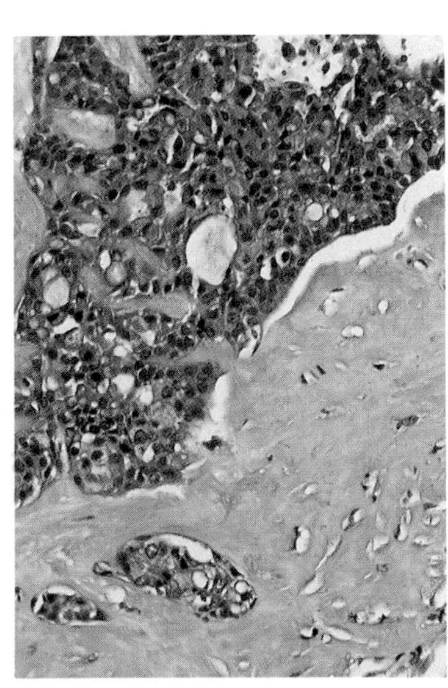

Fig. 253 Carcinoma in pleomorphic adenoma.

22 / Salivary gland cysts and chronic non-specific sialadenitis

Salivary gland cysts (mucoceles)

Mucous extravasation cysts

Most common type of soft tissue cyst. Minor glands, especially of the lip, are affected.

Aetiology

Probably mainly result from injury to the duct, leading to leakage and formation of pools of saliva in overlying soft tissues with inflammatory reaction (Fig. 254). Coalescence of pools of saliva leads to the formation of a cyst with lining of fibroblasts and compressed fibrous tissue (Figs 255 & 256).

Salivary retention cysts

Rare variant of mucocele produced by duct obstruction, forming a clinically similar lesion but the cyst is lined by flattened duct epithelium (Fig. 257).

Prognosis

Mucoceles respond to simple excision but the damaged gland must also be removed to prevent recurrence.

Chronic non-specific sialadenitis

Aetiology

Commonly a consequence of obstruction to salivary secretion, sometimes in association with calculus formation.

Microscopy

Scattered, mainly periductal infiltration by chronic inflammatory cells, dilatation of ducts, degeneration of acini and increasing fibrous replacement (see Fig. 258, p.148) are the characteristic features.

Prognosis

Chronically inflamed glands do not resolve spontaneously and need to be removed to exclude a tumour as the cause of the swelling.

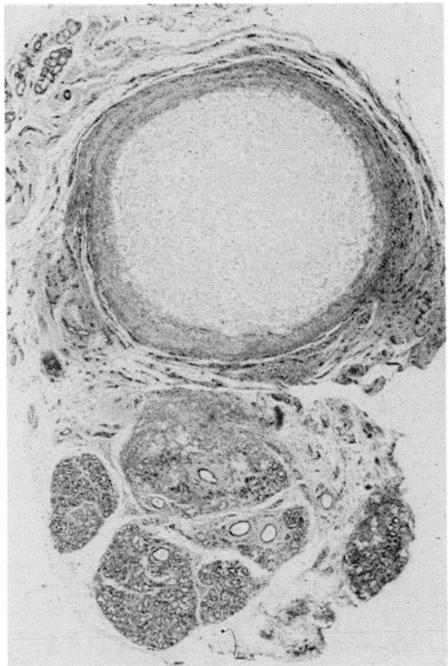

Fig. 254 Extravasation mucocele and attached salivary tissue.

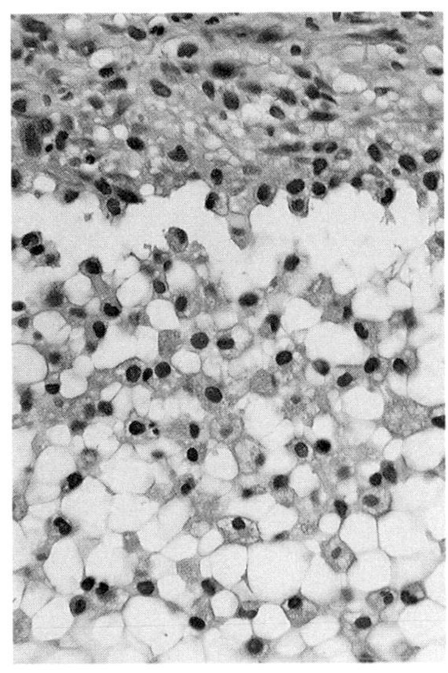

Fig. 255 Extravasation mucocele: connective tissue wall (above); mucin- and lipid-laden macrophages in contents.

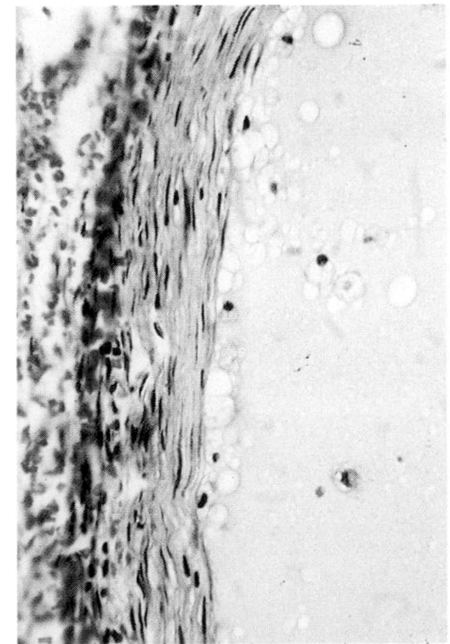

Fig. 256 Extravasation mucocele: fibrous wall.

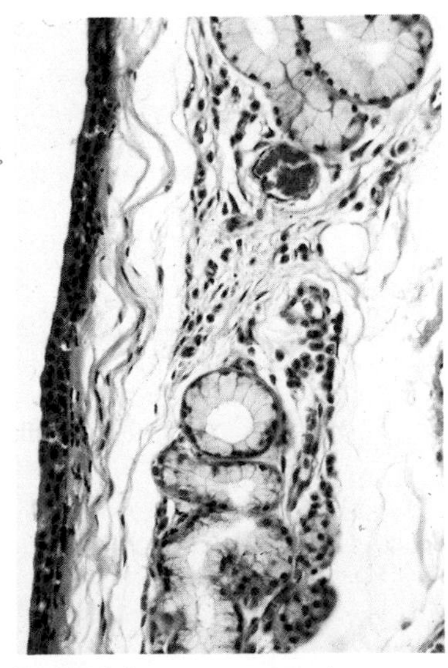

Fig. 257 Salivary mucous retention cyst: epithelial lining.

Salivary calculi

Calculi form usually by concretion of calcium salts round a nidus of organic matter, particularly in the submandibular gland. Calculi may be multiple within the gland or solitary and in the duct. Sialadenitis with duct dilatation is typically associated.

Microscopy

Calculi appear either as lamellated structures or multiple concretions which fuse to form a single mass. The surrounding duct epithelium may undergo squamous metaplasia (Fig. 259) and the surrounding tissue may be inflamed.

Prognosis

Calculi need to be removed as obstruction of the duct predisposes to infection of the gland.

Sjögren syndrome and related disorders

Sjögren syndrome comprises dry mouth, dry eyes and connective tissue disease—usually rheumatoid arthritis. Sicca syndrome has no associated connective tissue disease and differs in the immunological findings. Salivary lymphoepithelial lesion is the same histologically as Sjögren syndrome. These conditions mainly affect women, usually over 50.

Microscopy

Infiltration of salivary tissue by lymphocytes and plasma cells is initially periductal (Fig. 260). The infiltrate spreads outwards and leads to progressive destruction of acini but ducts are more resistant (Fig. 261). Eventually, only lymphoplasmacytic cells and islands of hyperplastic duct epithelium ('epimyoepithelial islands') may remain. The lymphoplasmacytic infiltrate remains confined within the salivary lobules and does not penetrate the gland septa.

Labial salivary glands show close correlation with the parotid changes, but epimyoepithelial islands are rare.

Prognosis

There is no curative treatment and lymphomatous change is a hazard. Symptomatic treatment is needed for xerostomia and xerophthalmia.

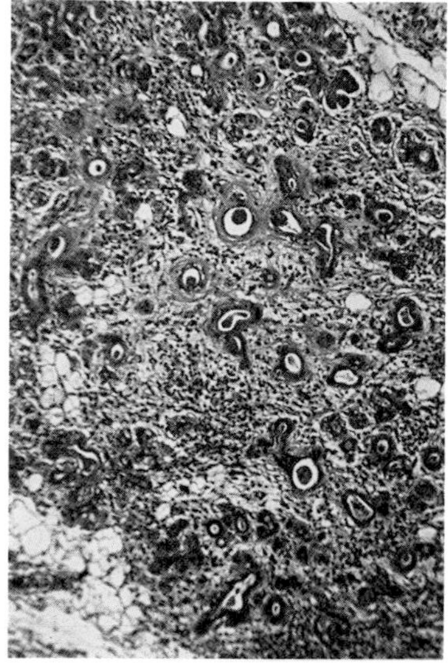

Fig. 258 Non-specific sialadenitis.

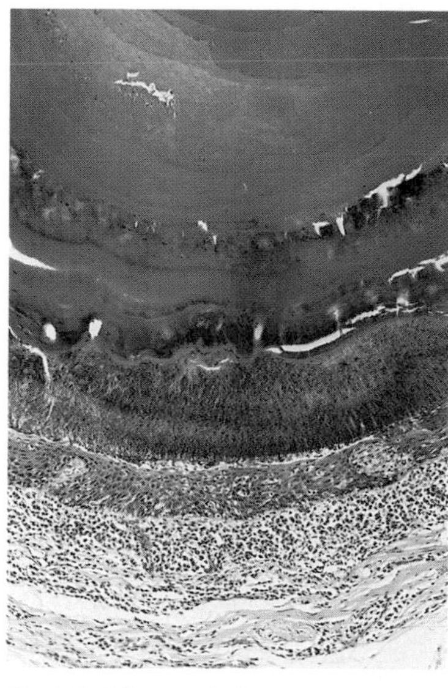

Fig. 259 Salivary calculi: squamous metaplasia of duct lining.

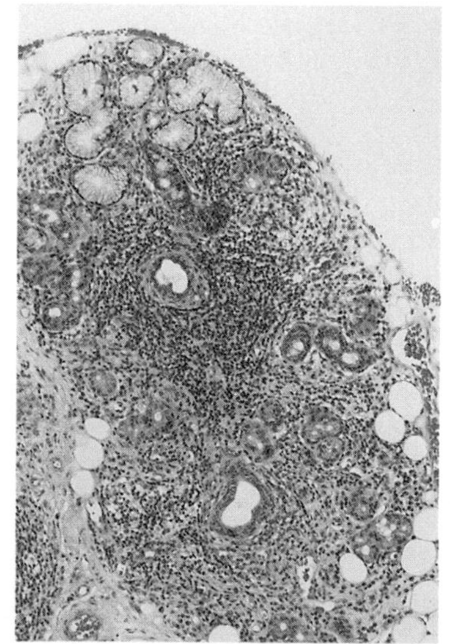

Fig. 260 Sjögren syndrome: early stage.

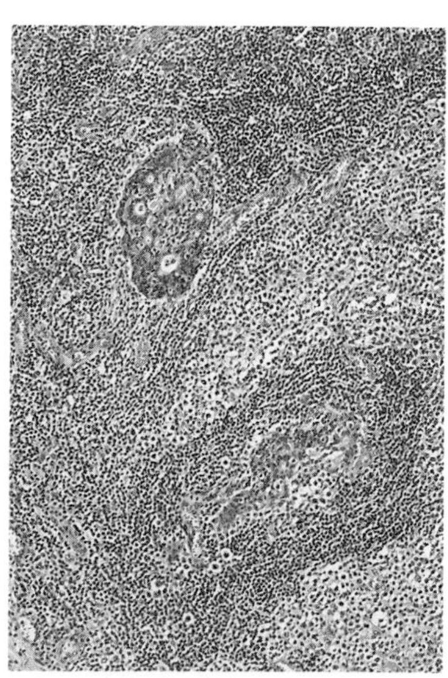

Fig. 261 Sjögren syndrome: destruction of gland acini, and epimyoepithelial islands.

23 / Granulomatous diseases

Histologically, granulomas are focal, rounded collections of macrophages, often with giant cells, as in tuberculosis. Clinically, however, 'granuloma' is used for many chronic inflammatory conditions (e.g. apical granuloma, etc.) which lack granulomas histologically.

Tuberculosis

Aetiology Tuberculous oral ulceration, secondary to chest infection, is occasionally seen in AIDS patients, otherwise very rare. Mycobacteria are rarely found in oral lesions but are present in sputum.

Microscopy Deep ulcer with overhanging edges (usually on dorsum of tongue) with tuberculous granulomas and Langhans' giant cells (Figs 262 & 263).

Prognosis Response depends on clearing the pulmonary infection. In AIDS patients the prognosis of mycobacterial infections is poor due to multiply resistant bacteria. In the absence of HIV infection, tuberculosis usually responds to multiagent chemotherapy.

Fungal infections (systemic mycoses)

Immunosuppressed and AIDS patients are susceptible to many fungal infections such as histoplasmosis or aspergillosis. Other such infections are common in South America. Many produce oral lesions at some stage.

Microscopy Several of the mycoses (*not* candidosis) produce granulomatous reactions more or less resembling tuberculosis (Fig. 264). Tissue forms of the fungus, usually spore forms or hyphae, may sometimes be detectable, but usually only with special stains. *Histoplasma capsulatum* is unusual in that the spores, with characteristic halo-like capsule, may be seen in H & E stained sections (Fig. 265).

Prognosis Treatment with amphotericin or an imidazole antifungal drug is likely to be effective unless infection is too widespread.

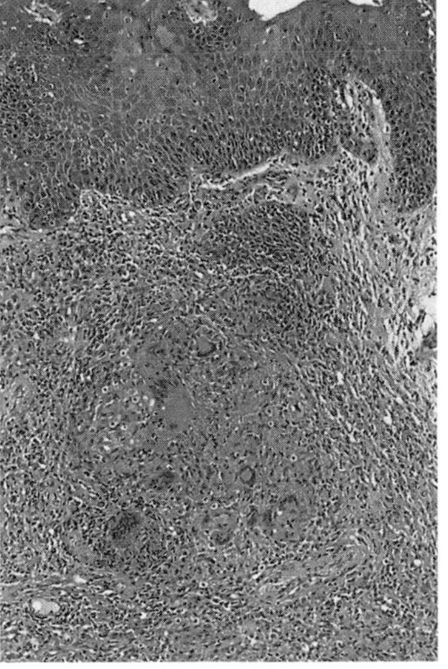

Fig. 262 Tuberculous ulcer of lip edge.

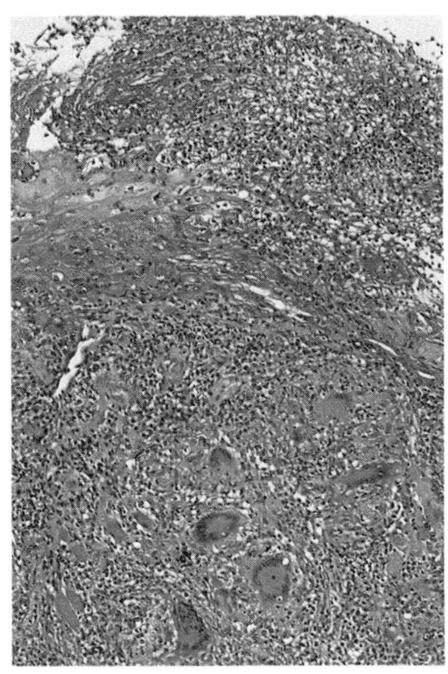

Fig. 263 Tuberculous granuloma beneath ulcer.

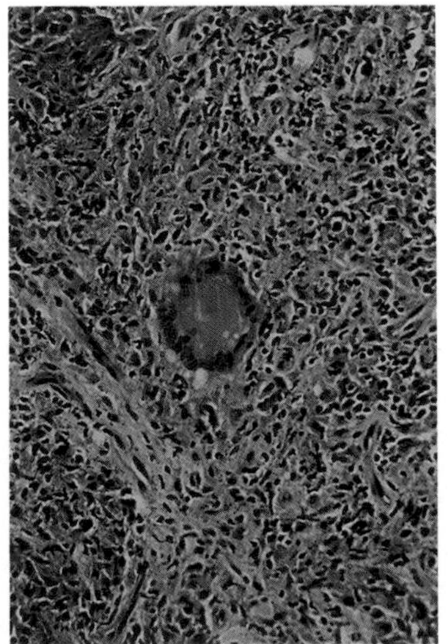

Fig. 264 Histoplasmosis of the tongue: Langhans giant cell and granuloma.

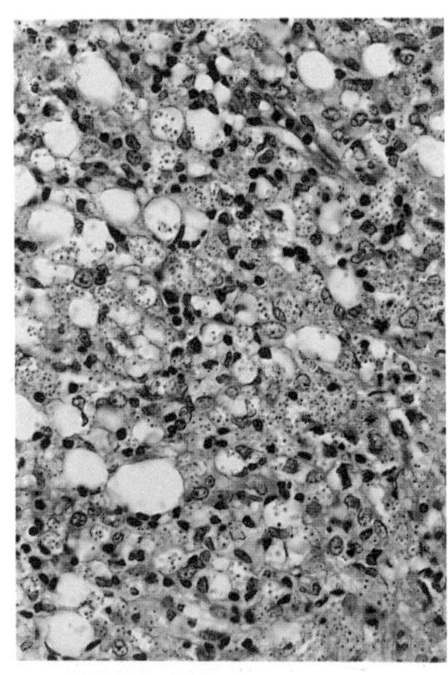

Fig. 265 *Histoplasma capsulatum*: spores surrounded by halo-like capsule.

Actinomycosis

Neither a mycosis nor a granulomatous disease histologically. Clinically, actinomycosis most frequently affects the soft tissues at the angle of the jaw, but only exceptionally rarely involves bone. The causative organism is usually *Actinomyces israelii*, a filamentous bacterium found in normal mouths. The reason for its occasional invasion of tissues in the immunocompetent person is unknown, but it is now increasingly rarely seen.

Microscopy

Actinomyces israelii, if it invades the tissues, produces multiple abscesses. There is suppuration, with a central colony of filamentous bacteria surrounded by fibrosis, and sinuses develop (Figs 266 & 267). Inflammatory reaction and fibrosis typically fail to localize the infection, which, if untreated, spreads through the tissues producing multiple sinuses. Lymph nodes are not involved except by direct extension of the infection.

The diagnosis is confirmed by culture of pus, but is unlikely to be positive unless 'sulphur granules' (colonies of Actinomyces) are present.

Prognosis

Good response to vigorous, early treatment, usually with penicillin. Surgical drainage rarely required.

Sarcoidosis

Aetiology

Unknown. Minor immunological defects may be associated—especially negative reaction to tuberculin.

Pathology

Hilar lymph nodes and sometimes peripheral lung are the main sites but almost any tissue can be affected. There is a predilection also for salivary tissue, especially labial glands. Gingival enlargement develops in some cases.

Microscopy

Compact histiocytic granulomas without caseation, often multiple and with giant cells (Fig. 268).

Diagnosis

Diagnosis is usually dependent on combined laboratory and clinical findings, in particular, evidence of pulmonary involvement, biopsy of affected tissue, positive Kveim test or raised serum angiotensin converting enzyme (ACE) levels. ➡

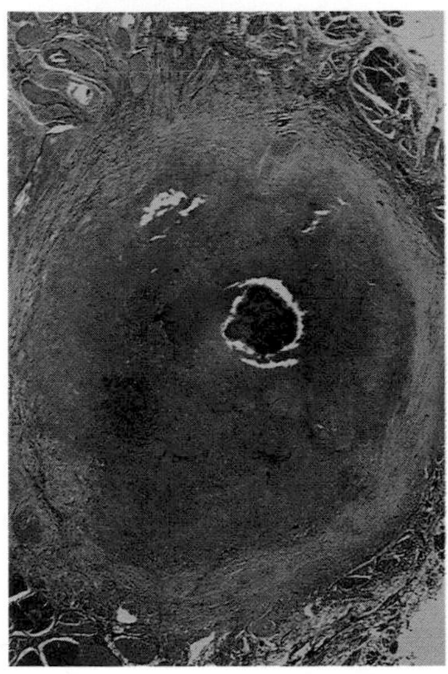

Fig. 266 Actinomycosis: loculus with central colony surrounded by neutrophils and fibrous abscess wall.

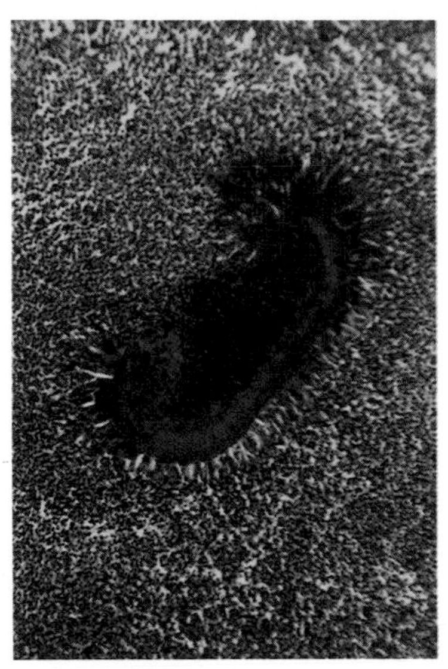

Fig. 267 Actinomycosis: detail of bacterial colony.

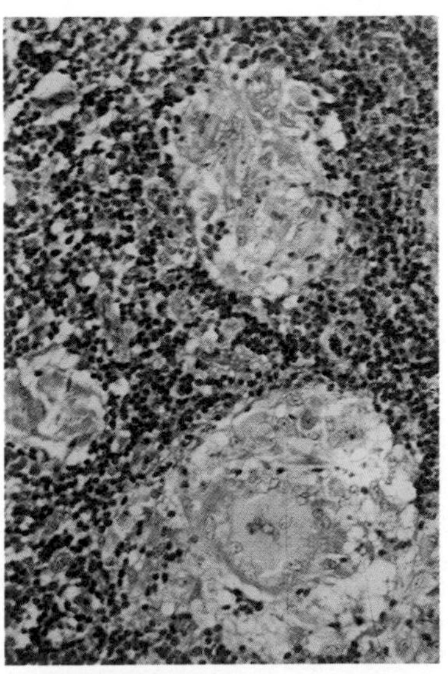

Fig. 268 Sarcoidosis: typical granuloma with giant cell.

Sarcoidosis (cont'd)

Heerfordt syndrome comprises swelling of the parotid glands, xerostomia, uveitis and facial palsy.

Prognosis

Intralesional corticosteroids are sometimes given for troublesome oral lesions. Pulmonary fibrosis or hypercalcaemia are the main complications for which systemic corticosteroids are required.

Crohn's disease

Aetiology unknown. Typically there is intestinal (particularly ileocaecal) granulomatous inflammation, causing ulceration, fibrosis and thickening of the intestinal wall and bowel dysfunction (diarrhoea and/or constipation and pain). Complications include malabsorption leading to vitamin deficiencies.

Oral lesions consist of soft mucosal thickenings causing a cobblestone appearance, mucosal tags or ulceration.

Microscopy

Subepithelial oedema, chronic inflammation and granulomas which are typically loose-textured, scattered and sometimes present only deeply (Figs 269 & 270).

Prognosis

Investigation is required for bowel symptoms which may respond to sulphasalazine or its analogues but response is variable. Oral lesions sometimes respond to sulphasalazine.

Melkersson Rosenthal syndrome

Characterized by facial or labial swelling, recurrent facial palsy and fissured tongue. Unknown aetiology. Shows granulomas in the affected tissues.

Orofacial granulomatosis

This term is used for granulomatous lesions clinically and histologically resembling those of Crohn's disease or sarcoidosis but without any other features of such diseases. Some of these reactions appear to be due to food additives and occasionally respond to restriction diets. In others, manifestations of sarcoidosis or Crohn's disease may appear later (Fig. 271).

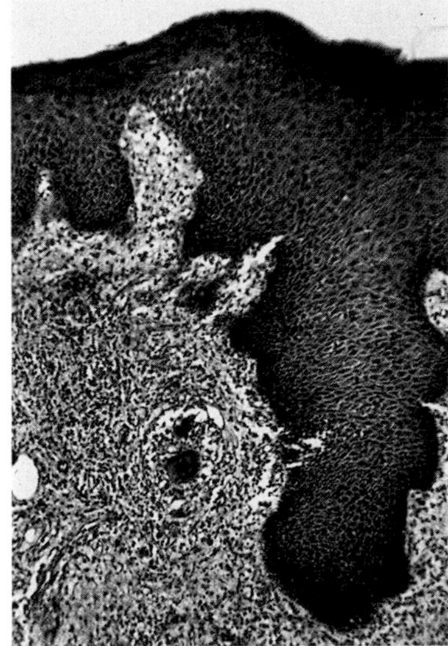

Fig. 269 Crohn's disease of oral mucosa.

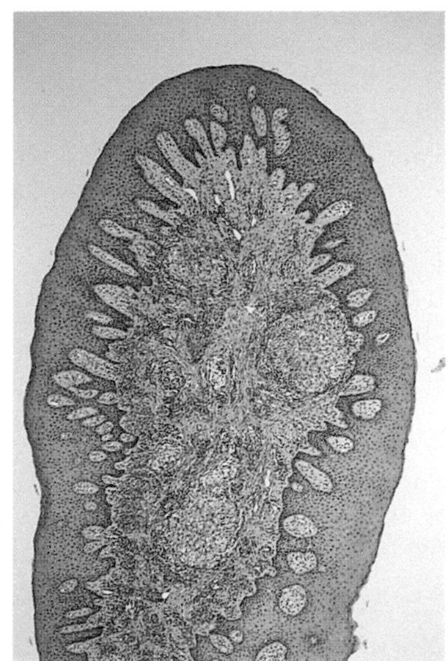

Fig. 270 Crohn's disease: a mucosal tag containing granulomas.

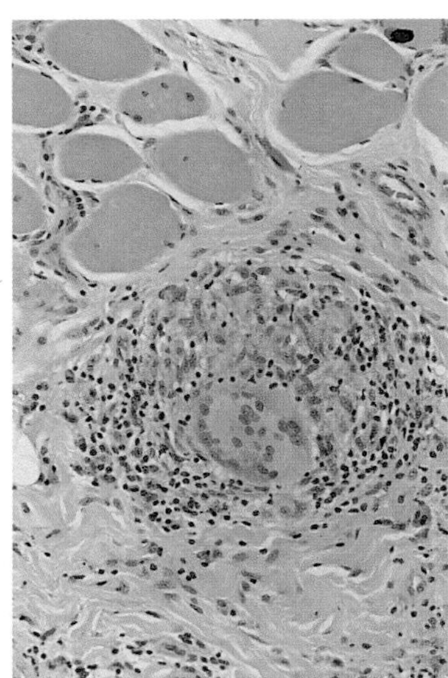

Fig. 271 Orofacial granulomatosis. Similar granulomas to Crohn's disease in the absence of systemic disease.

Midline granuloma syndrome (lethal midline granuloma)

These rare syndromes have initial nasopharyngeal symptoms leading to midfacial destruction of tissues and a fatal termination. In the past, similar appearances could be produced by such diseases as tuberculosis, syphilis or systemic mycoses, but these are separate and treatable entities. The main causes of midline granuloma are now Wegener's granulomatosis and peripheral T-cell lymphomas.

Wegener's granulomatosis

Typically comprises granulomatous nasal inflammation, pulmonary and renal involvement, plus, occasionally, a characteristic proliferative gingivitis ('strawberry gums') or, later, mucosal ulceration.

Microscopy

There is necrotizing arteritis with giant cells (Fig. 272) scattered or related to the inflamed vessels. The giant cells may be small with few nuclei or resemble Langhans cells. Granulomas are a characteristic feature but may be difficult to see in a dense inflammatory infiltrate.

Gingival biopsy showing giant cells may allow early successful cytotoxic treatment. Otherwise renal involvement can be fatal.

Nasopharyngeal T-cell lymphomas

Nasopharyngeal T-cell lymphomas can produce initial symptoms indistinguishable from Wegener's granulomatosis but, occasionally, extension of tissue destruction produces palatal perforation and ulceration (Fig. 273).

Microscopy

The cellular picture is highly pleomorphic but the lymphoma cells can surround, infiltrate and destroy blood vessels and so closely mimic true (inflammatory) vasculitis.

Prognosis

Ultimately systemic spread is like that of other lymphomas but may be slow. Early cytotoxic treatment and/or radiotherapy may be effective.

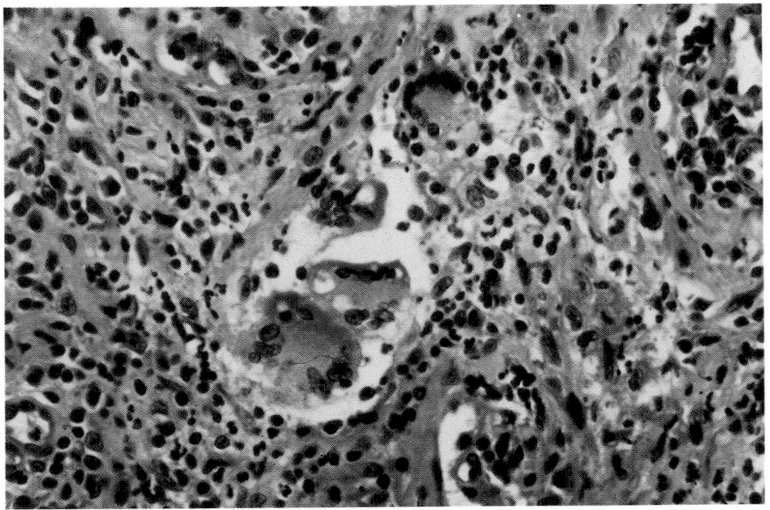

Fig. 272 Wegener's granulomatosis: typical giant cells in gingival biopsy.

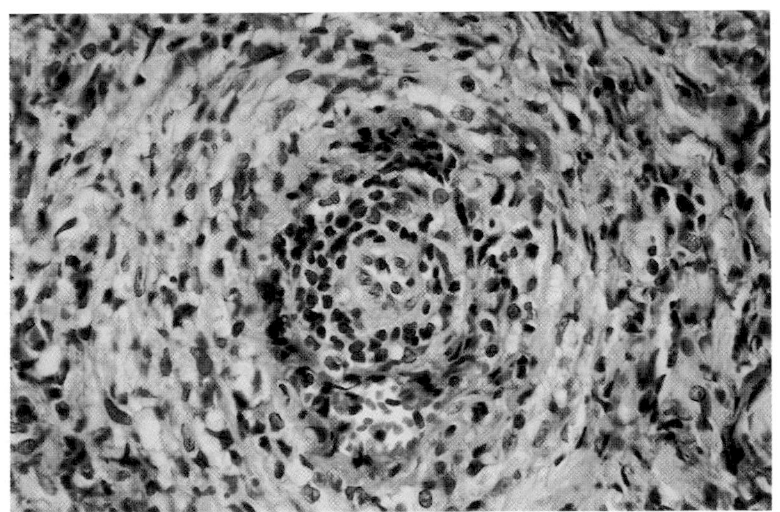

Fig. 273 Nasopharyngeal T-cell lymphoma: neoplastic lymphocytes surrounding and destroying an arteriole.

24 / Miscellaneous fibrotic conditions

Progressive systemic sclerosis (scleroderma)

Aetiology

A connective tissue (autoimmune) disease producing progressive fibrosis and stiffening of the skin and viscera. Limitation of opening of the mouth and movement of the tongue and Sjögren syndrome may develop. Antinuclear bodies are present.

Microscopy

Progressive fibrous thickening of submucosa extending into and destroying superficial muscle fibres. There is a perivascular lymphocytic infiltrate (Fig. 274).

Prognosis

The 5-year survival rate is only about 50% due to visceral or pulmonary disease.

Oral submucous fibrosis

Aetiology

Affects those from the Indian subcontinent and may be related to Areca nut chewing, but the aetiology is uncertain. It is not an autoimmune condition. There is intense, symmetrical, thick board-like stiffening of sites such as the palate, cheeks or lip, but not of the viscera or other parts of the body.

Microscopy

Similar to scleroderma but more intense and lacking perivascular infiltrate (Fig. 275). Sometimes there is epithelial dysplasia, which is possibly premalignant.

Prognosis

Oral submucous fibrosis is disabling when it becomes impossible to open the mouth adequately. There is also a risk of carcinomatous change.

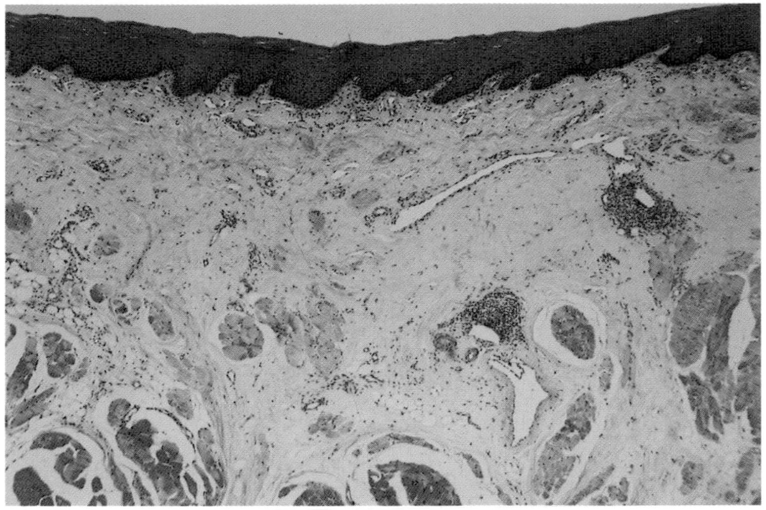

Fig. 274 Scleroderma: submucosal fibrosis with muscle destruction in the tongue and perivascular lymphocytic infiltrate.

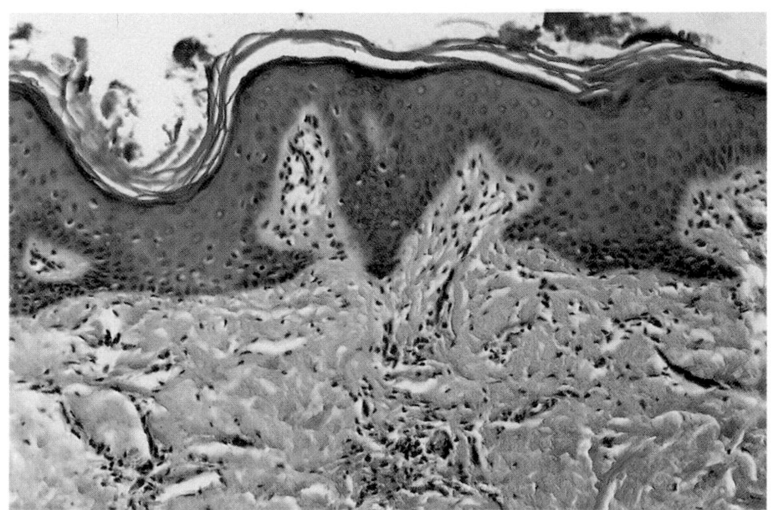

Fig. 275 Oral submucous fibrosis: deeper extension of fibrosis and muscle destruction than in scleroderma.

25 / HIV infection and AIDS

Human immunodeficiency virus (HIV) particularly infects and destroys T helper (CD4) lymphocytes, leading (usually) to progressively more severe defects, particularly of cell-mediated immunity and, eventually, gross immunodeficiency. Death is usually due to opportunistic infections but lymphomas and Kaposi's sarcoma (see p. 123) are also common. CNS cells are also directly involved and cranial nerve lesions may result.

'Hairy' leukoplakia

Usually painless, soft, white plaque with corrugated surface along lateral borders of the tongue. Hair-like protrusions of keratin are rarely seen.

Microscopy

Hyperkeratosis with ridged surface (Fig. 276); often colonized by *C. albicans* or bacteria. A zone of koilocytes (vacuolated and ballooned prickle cells with pyknotic nuclei) is seen in the prickle cell layer (Fig. 277). Epstein–Barr virus capsid antigen is identifiable in the nuclei (Fig. 278).

Prognosis

There is no evidence of malignant potential but over 80% of these patients develop AIDS within 3 years.

Other typical oral manifestations

- Candidosis (any type)
- HIV gingivitis or periodontitis
- Necrotizing ulcerative gingivitis
- Kaposi's sarcoma and lymphomas

  Less frequent are:
- atypical ulcerations
- lymphoepithelial lesions of salivary glands
- infections by herpes simplex or varicella-zoster, cytomegalovirus or human papillomavirus
- deep mycoses.

See preceding pages for the pathology of these lesions.

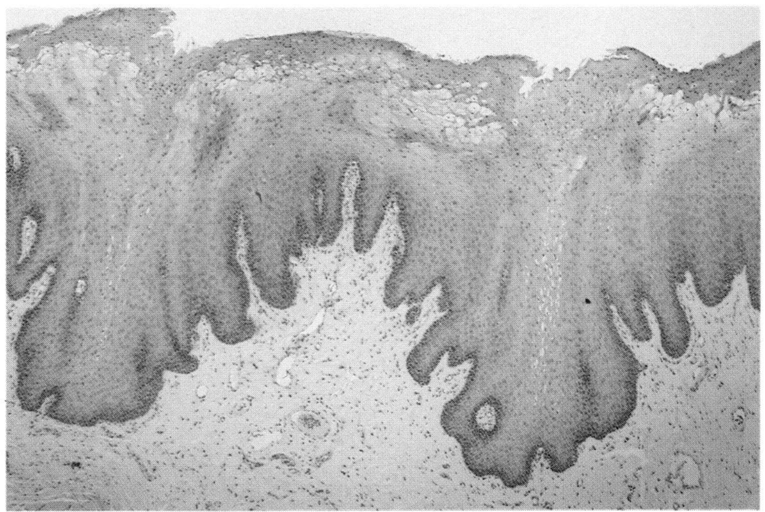

Fig. 276 Hairy leukoplakia in HIV infection: ridged, hyperkeratotic surface; acanthosis and scanty inflammatory infiltrate beneath.

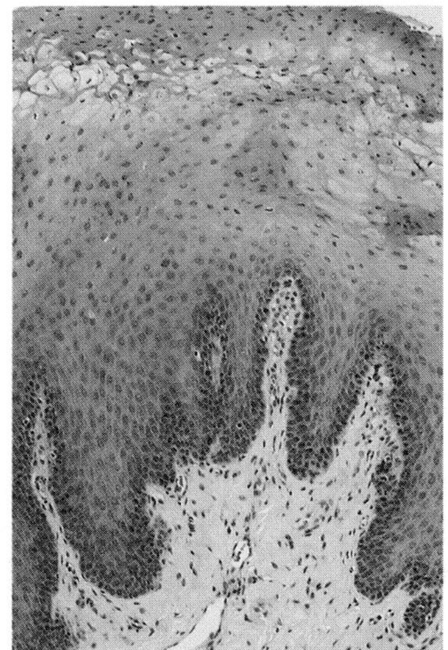

Fig. 277 Hairy leukoplakia: hyperplastic epithelium with koilocytes beneath the surface.

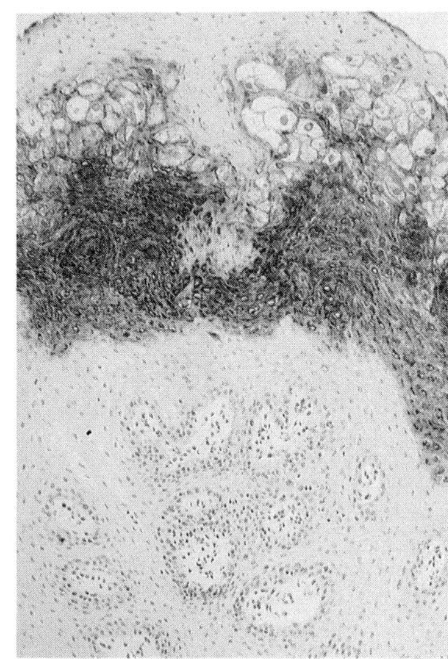

Fig. 278 Hairy leukoplakia: positive staining for Epstein–Barr virus capsid antigen.

Index